Art and Challenges Involved in the Treatment of Ischaemic Damage

*Edited by Nieves Saiz-Sapena,
Fernando Aparici-Robles and Georgios Tsoulfas*

Published in London, United Kingdom

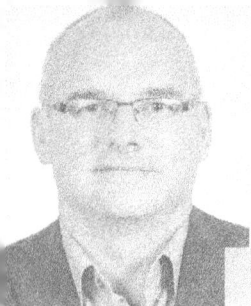
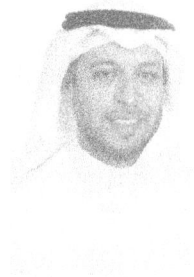
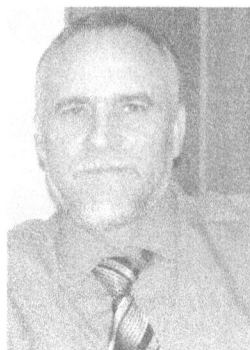
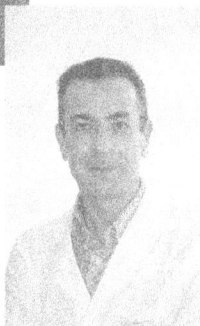
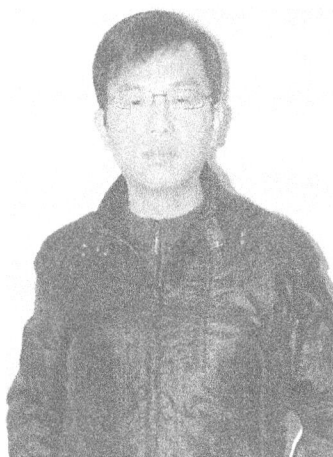
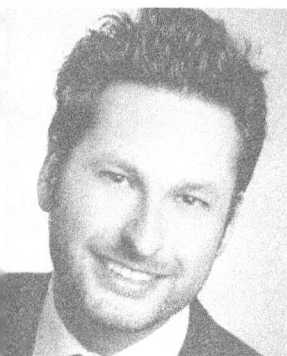
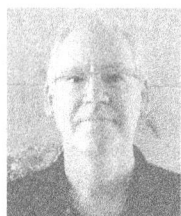

IntechOpen

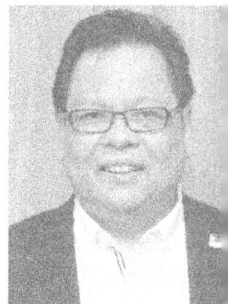
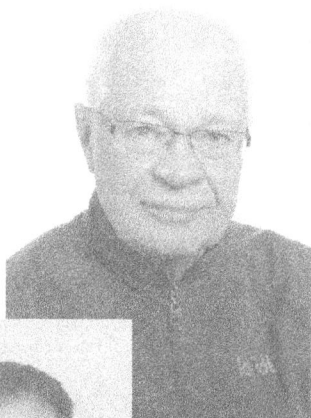
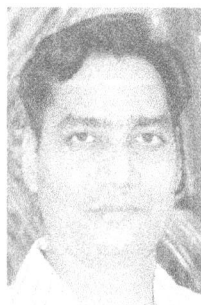
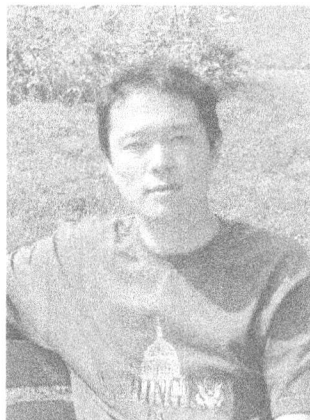
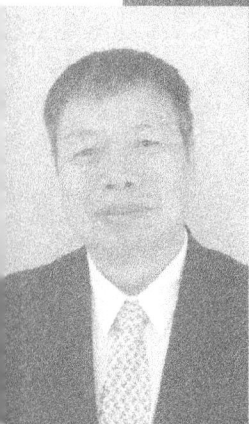
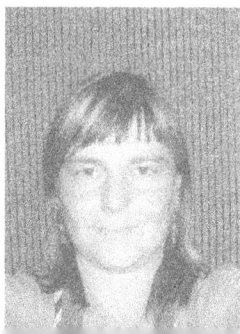

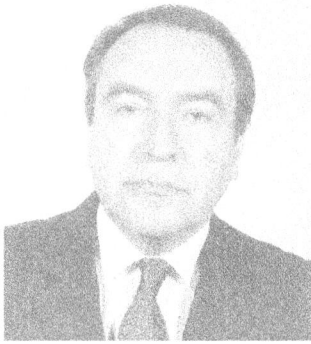

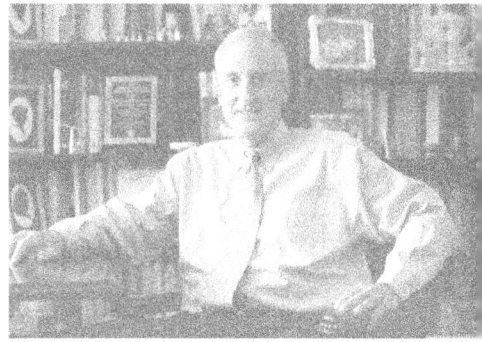

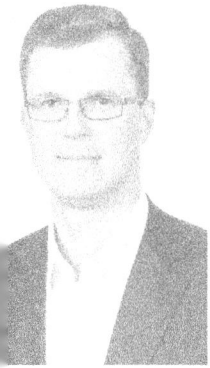

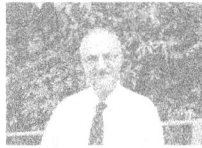

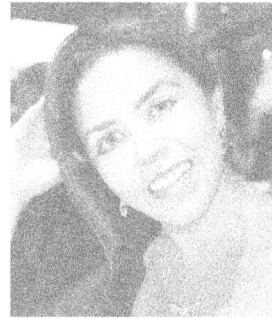

Supporting open minds since 2005

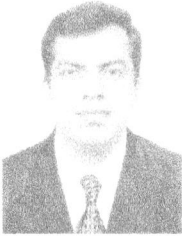

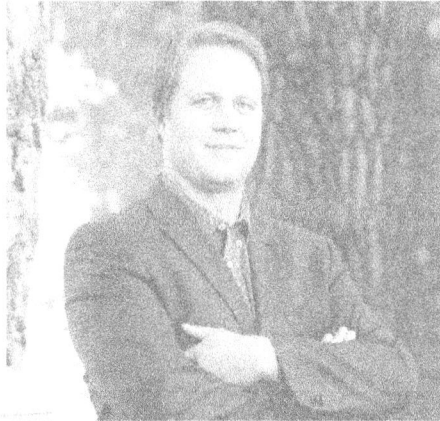

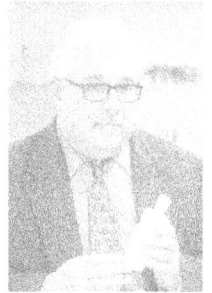

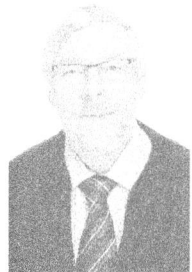

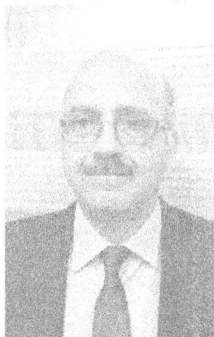

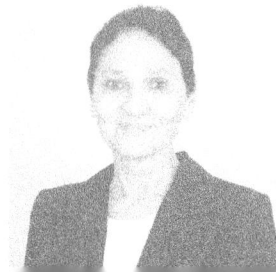

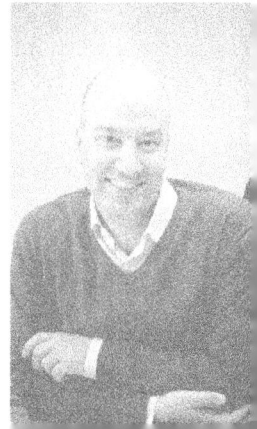

Art and Challenges Involved in the Treatment of Ischaemic Damage
http://dx.doi.org/10.5772/intechopen.94682
Edited by Nieves Saiz-Sapena, Fernando Aparici-Robles and Georgios Tsoulfas

Contributors
Prasanna Venkatesh Ramesh, Shruthy Vaishali Ramesh, Prajnya Ray, Aji Kunnath Devadas, Tensingh Joshua, Anugraha Balamurugan, Meena Kumari Ramesh, Ramesh Rajasekaran, G. Ravi Kiran, Chih-Hsin Hsu, Po-Sheng Chen, Jia-Ling Lin, Po-Kai Yang, Adam Raskin, Kofi Ansah, Anil Verma, Hisham Badreldin, Omar Alshaya, Khalid Bin Saleh, Abdulrahman Alshaya, Mohammed Aldhaeefi, Pinar Gelener, Süha Halil Akpinar, Mu-Yang Hsieh, Daniel Brandão, Flavia H. Feier, Melina U. Melere, Antonio N. Kalil, Alex Horbe

Notice
Statements and opinions expressed in the chapters are these of the individual contributors and not necessarily those of the editors or publisher. No responsibility is accepted for the accuracy of information contained in the published chapters. The publisher assumes no responsibility for any damage or injury to persons or property arising out of the use of any materials, instructions, methods or ideas contained in the book.

First published in London, United Kingdom, 2022 by IntechOpen
IntechOpen is the global imprint of INTECHOPEN LIMITED, registered in England and Wales, registration number: 11086078, 5 Princes Gate Court, London, SW7 2QJ, United Kingdom
Printed in Croatia

British Library Cataloguing-in-Publication Data
A catalogue record for this book is available from the British Library

Additional hard and PDF copies can be obtained from orders@intechopen.com

Art and Challenges Involved in the Treatment of Ischaemic Damage
Edited by Nieves Saiz-Sapena, Fernando Aparici-Robles and Georgios Tsoulfas
p. cm.
Print ISBN 978-1-83969-785-2
Online ISBN 978-1-83969-786-9
eBook (PDF) ISBN 978-1-83969-787-6

We are IntechOpen,
the world's leading publisher of
Open Access books
Built by scientists, for scientists

6,000+
Open access books available

148,000+
International authors and editors

185M+
Downloads

Our authors are among the

156
Countries delivered to

Top 1%
most cited scientists

12.2%
Contributors from top 500 universities

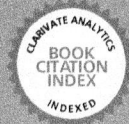

Interested in publishing with us?
Contact book.department@intechopen.com

Numbers displayed above are based on latest data collected.
For more information visit www.intechopen.com

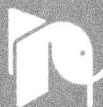

Meet the editors

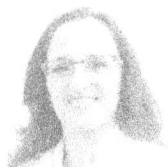

Dr. Nieves Saiz-Sapena, MD, Ph.D., is an anesthesiologist at Hospital General Universitario de Valencia, Spain. She has more than twenty-five years of experience in anesthesia in specialized fields such as neurosurgery, airway management, hostile environments, and bariatric surgery. She has numerous publications to her credit and is a member of several national and international scientific societies. Dr. Saiz-Sapena has taught at various institutions in Spain, including Universidad de Navarra, Universidad de Barcelona, Universidad Cardenal Herrera-CEU, and Universidad Catolica de Valencia, both on-site and online.

Fernando Aparici-Robles is a Doctor of Medicine and Surgery from the University of Valencia and obtained his Ph.D. at the University of Valencia, Spain. He has over 20 years of professional experience, especially in interventional neuroradiology. He is the head of the Neuroradiology Section at the Hospital Universitario y Politecnico La Fe, Valencia, Spain. He has participated in the launch and implementation of the Stroke program in Valencia County, which includes thrombectomy procedures. He is an associate professor at the University of Valencia, and formerly an associate professor at Universidad Catolica San Vicente Martir, Valencia. Currently, he is an active member of several scientific societies including ECR, ASNR, and CIRSE, especially involved in Neurointerventional Sections. He also plays a role as a reviewer in a number of national and international scientific journals. Another field he is involved in is education, as the coordinator of the specialist training in Radiology at the Hospital Universitario y Politecnico La Fe.

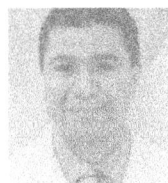

Dr. Georgios Tsoulfas received his medical degree from Brown University School of Medicine, Rhode Island, and completed his general surgery residency at the University of Iowa Hospitals and Clinics, as well as a transplant research fellowship at the Starzl Transplant Institute, University of Pittsburgh. He then completed a two-year transplantation surgery fellowship at Massachusetts General Hospital, Harvard Medical School, and then joined the Division of Solid Organ Transplantation and Hepatobiliary Surgery at the University of Rochester Medical Center, New York, as an assistant professor of surgery. He has currently moved back to Greece, where he is a professor of Transplantation Surgery and chief of the Department of Transplantation Surgery at the Aristotle University School of Medicine. He has published more than 150 papers in peer-reviewed journals and PubMed, as well as 35 book chapters. He is a reviewer for more than forty international journals and serves on the editorial boards of several others.

Contents

Preface

This edited volume *Art and Challenges Involved in the Treatment of Ischaemic Damage* is a collection of reviewed and relevant research chapters, concerning the developments within the field of study.

The book includes scholarly contributions by various authors and is edited by a group of experts pertinent to this specific field.

Each contribution comes as a separate chapter complete in itself but directly related to the book's topics and objectives.

The edited volume includes chapters dealing with the topics:

Direct Oral Anticoagulants and Vitamin K Antagonists: Role in Thrombotic Damage, Safety, and Indications

Recent Advances in Thrombolysis and Thrombectomy in Acute Ischemic Stroke Treatment: Neurologist's and Interventional Neuroradiologist's Perspective

Endovascular Treatment for Acute Mesenteric Ischemia

Choosing the Right Guidewire: The Key for a Successful Revascularization

Revascularization Strategies in Liver Transplantation

The Holistic Spectrum of Thrombotic Ocular Complications: Recent Advances with Diagnosis, Prevention, and Management Guidelines

Management of Pulmonary Thromboembolism

Advances of Thrombectomy in Venous Thromboembolism

Mechanical Thrombectomy for Acute Pulmonary Ischemia

The target audience comprises scholars, practicing researchers, academics, Ph.D. students, and other scientists.

IntechOpen

Direct Oral Anticoagulants and Vitamin K Antagonists: Role in Thrombotic Damage, Safety, and Indications

Mohammed Aldhaeefi, Abdulrahman Alshaya,
Khalid Bin Saleh, Omar Alshaya and Hisham Badreldin

Abstract

This chapter is intended to discuss the available oral anticoagulants, including vitamin K antagonists and the Direct Oral Anticoagulants such as dabigatran, apixaban, rivaroxaban, and edoxaban. It will review their basic pharmacology, pharmacokinetics, pharmacodynamics, dosage forms, clinical indications, and place in therapy. Finally, this chapter will also discuss the currently available reversal agents.

Keywords: anticoagulants, vitamin K antagonists, direct oral anticoagulants, reversal agents

1. Introduction

Thromboembolic diseases are a leading source of morbidity and death in the United States. Thrombosis can happen in either the arteries or the veins. Acute myocardial infarction (MI), ischemic stroke, and limb gangrene are all caused by arterial thrombosis. Deep vein thrombosis (DVT), which can cause post-thrombotic syndrome, and pulmonary embolism (PE), which can be fatal or cause thromboembolic pulmonary hypertension, are both examples of venous thromboembolism (VTE). Arterial thrombosis is usually managed using antiplatelet therapy. On the other hand, VTE episodes are typically managed using anticoagulant therapy [1].

Anticoagulant drugs are the mainstay of therapy for many thrombotic disorders. The selection of one agent over the other is usually guided by balancing the risks versus the benefits of these anticoagulants. Also, it requires deep knowledge and understanding of the clinical pharmacology, efficacy, safety, and clinical outcomes for each of these anticoagulants.

Historically. Jay McLean and William Henry Howell discovered heparin a century ago, in 1914. However, it was first used in clinical practice in the 1940s. It's given subcutaneously or intravenously, and it binds to antithrombin. This will improve its capacity to inactivate several clotting factors such as thrombin, factor Xa, and factor IXa [2]. Later on, several oral and parenteral antithrombotic agents are used to prevent and treat thrombotic episodes. In 1940, Karl Link and colleagues discovered warfarin which is a vitamin-k antagonist. Warfarin was first marketed as a rodenticide. Later on, it was adopted for therapeutic usage as an anticoagulant [3].

In 2003, the discovery of ximelagatran showed that a particular oral thrombin inhibitor might be safe and effective in a range of thrombotic diseases, paving the way for introducing a new class of anticoagulants [4]. Following these advancements, a major millstone was declared in the field of anticoagulation. Several direct oral anticoagulants (DOACs) targeting factors Xa and II were introduced from 2007 to 2014. According to several landmark randomized studies, they were shown to be equally safe and efficacious as warfarin in preventing and treating venous thromboembolism and stroke prevention in atrial fibrillation. These advancements led to an enormous change in the landscape of managing thrombotic events [5].

This chapter is intended to review the currently available oral anticoagulants, including vitamin K antagonists (VKA), such as warfarin, and the (DOACs) such as dabigatran, apixaban, rivaroxaban, and edoxaban. In addition, it will discuss periprocedural management of anticoagulants, reversal modalities and highlight the major future advancements in the field of anticoagulation.

2. Vitamin K Antagonists

Warfarin is a vitamin K antagonist that was approved by the US Food and Drug Authority (FDA) in 1954 for stroke prevention. It is approved in many other indications such as managing and preventing VTE. Until recently, it was the only oral agent approved for these indications. However, more oral anticoagulants have been approved that possess more advantages and better pharmacokinetic properties. However, warfarin still a widely used medication to prevent blood clotting disorders. Warfarin administration remains a challenge despite being used for more than 60 years. Warfarin has a narrow therapeutic index and monitored regularly using international normalized ratio (INR). Duo to it inter and intra individual variation in response and multiple drug and food interactions, warfarin was replaced as a first line anticoagulant agent [6].

2.1 Mechanism of action

Warfarin exerts it anticoagulant effect by interfering with vitamin K epoxide reductase in the liver which serve as a cofactor for the carboxylation of glutamate to γ-carboxyglutamates. This process leads to the inhibition of vitamin K–dependent γ-carboxylation of factors II, VII, IX, and X. However, Vitamin K antagonist does not inhibit the existing γ-carboxyglutamates that can lead to delay in its anticoagulant effect [6].

2.2 Pharmacology

Warfarin consists of a racemic mixture of S-warfarin and R-warfarin, in which the S- form being more active. It has high bioavailability with rapid absorption from the gastrointestinal tract. After drug administration, warfarin reaches maximum concentration within 90 mins. Warfarin is highly albumin bound with a half-life of 36–42 hours. Warfarin is metabolized mainly in the liver through the cytochrome P450 (CYP) enzymes. However, the two isomers and metabolized through a different pathway in the liver. CYP2C9 is associated with the metabolism of the more potent S-warfarin whereas R-warfarin mainly metabolized by CYP1A2 and CYP3A4 [6].

2.3 Indication and dosing

Warfarin has multiple indications including venous thrombosis, prosthetic heart valves and more commonly arterial fibrillation. Usually, the starting dose for warfarin is 5–10 mg daily. However, lower doses can be initiated for patients at high risk of bleeding. Patients with known genetic polymorphism in CYP2C9 or VKORC1 can be more sensitive to warfarin. Also, elderly patients, patients with chronic kidney disease or patients on other medications that can cause bleeding can be initiated at a lower dose and up titrated to INR goal. Duo to its delayed antithrombotic effect, patients with established clot or high risk for thrombosis are bridged with a fast-acting parenteral anticoagulant. Commonly, heparin or enoxaparin are given concomitantly with warfarin until INR is at goal for 2 consecutive days with a minimum of 5 days on parenteral anticoagulant [6].

2.4 Monitoring

Warfarin is a drug known for its narrow therapeutic index as well as having multiple drug and food interactions. Therefore, continuous monitoring is important to ensure anticoagulation efficacy is achieved and severe side effects are avoided. INR is calculated from prothrombin time which is a test that measures how long a clot is formed in a blood sample is performed when patients are on warfarin. Mostly, warfarin is given to achieve an INR goal of 2–3. However, patients with a mechanical mitral valves or mechanical aortic valve replacement with Starr-Edwards or disc valves have a higher INR target of 2.5–3.5 duo to higher thromboembolic risk [6].

2.5 Side effects

One of the major risks associated with using warfarin is bleeding and the severity of bleeding can vary. Majority of bleeding side effect is seen when INR supratherapeutic. Therefore, INR monitored and maintained at target is essential to minimize bleeding risk. There are several approaches to manage a supratherapeutic INR and the choice usually depends on the present or absent of bleeding, severity of bleeding and magnitude in which INR increased. Skin necrosis is a rare complication associated with warfarin administration in patients with protein C or S deficiency [6].

2.6 Drug interaction

Warfarin can interact with large number of medications. Drugs can cause pharmacodynamic or pharmacokinetic interaction with warfarin. Pharmacokinetic interactions involve medications that inhibit or induce CYP2C9, CYP1A2 or CYP3A4 which can alter warfarin concentration. Inhibitors of the CYP enzymes can interfere with warfarin metabolism that leads to higher warfarin concentration. However, CYP enzyme inducers can increase warfarin removal, therefore, decrease its effect. Pharmacodynamic interaction can occur when warfarin given with other anticoagulants, antiplatelet, non-steroidal anti-inflammatory drugs, or serotonin Reuptake Inhibitors. In which, these drugs can increase risk of bleeding [6].

3. Direct Oral Anticoagulants

Direct oral anticoagulants (DOACs) have been introduced to the market initially in 2010 as a potential alternative for warfarin. They possess many advantages over warfarin that placed them as the first-line anticoagulant option for many indications. These agents include apixaban, rivaroxaban, edoxaban, and dabigatran. All of these agents do not require regular monitoring of their anticoagulant effect and they achieve the target anticoagulation level shortly given their fast onset of action compared to warfarin. These significant advantages placed these agents as the preferred anticoagulant option by patients and clinicians [7].

3.1 Mechanism of action

Factor Xa is a crucial coagulation factor in the coagulation cascade that leads to the formation of thrombin and clot generation. Apixaban, rivaroxaban, and edoxaban, bind directly and reversibly to factor Xa and inhibit its action leading to a strong anticoagulation activity. On the other side, dabigatran inhibits directly factor IIa (thrombin), leading to the prevention of clot formation [8].

3.2 Pharmacology

Apixaban binds directly to factor Xa when free and when thrombin bound. It has a bioavailability of approximately 50% and reaches a plasma peak in about 2 hours with maximum plasma concentration in about 3 to 4 hours. It has a half-life of approximately 12 hours after oral administration necessitating twice-daily dosing. It is metabolized mainly by CYP3A4 and eliminated in both urine and feces. Renal elimination accounts for 27% of total clearance. Apixaban has no interaction with food but is a substrate of P-glycoprotein (P-gp) and CYP3A4 requiring vigilant review of concurrent medications for possible drug–drug interactions [9].

Dabigatran is the active form of the prodrug dabigatran etexilate, which binds thrombin directly and competitively inhibiting its activity. The approximate bioavailability of dabigatran after oral administration is 3–7%, with peak plasma concentration achievement within 2 hours. The bioavailability increased to 75% after the pellets were taken without the capsule. Therefore, the capsules should not be broken, chewed, or opened before administration. The half-life of dabigatran is approximately 12–17 hours, necessitating twice-daily dosing. Dabigatran is mainly eliminated in the urine with a renal clearance of roughly 80%. It is a substrate of P-gp and therefore, it carries a risk for drug–drug interactions [9].

Edoxaban binds selectively to factor Xa and inhibits its action without the need for a cofactor (i.e., antithrombin III). It has a bioavailability of approximately 62% and reaches a peak plasma concentration in about 1 to 2 hours. It has a half-life of approximately 10–14 hours, and 50% of the total clearance is through urine. Therefore, edoxaban blood levels are increased or decreased in patients with poor or good renal function. Edoxaban is a substrate for P-gp and CYP3A4, increasing the risk for drug–drug interactions [9].

Rivaroxaban is a selective inhibitor of factor Xa with no requirement for a cofactor (i.e., antithrombin III) with no direct effect on platelet aggregation. It has a very high bioavailability following oral administration of 2.5 mg and 10 mg doses reaching 80–100%. Administration with food increases the bioavailability of rivaroxaban. Therefore, it should be taken with food. Peak plasma concentration is achieved in about 2 to 4 hours. It has a renal clearance of up to 30%. Rivaroxaban is a substrate for P-gp increasing the risk of drug–drug interactions [9]. **Table 1** summarizes the pharmacological properties of DOACs.

3.3 Indications and dosing

DOACs are currently used in different indications, including reducing the incidence of stroke in patients with NVAF, treatment of acute VTE, and reducing

	Apixaban	Dabigatran	Edoxaban	Rivaroxaban
Mechanism of action	Factor Xa	Thrombin	Factor Xa	Factor Xa
Pro-drug	No	Yes	No	No
Bioavailability	50%	3%-7%	62%	66%-80%
Time to peak	2 hours	2 hours	1-2 hours	2-4 hours
Half-life	12 hours	12-17 hours	12-14 hours	9-13 hours
Protein binding	87%	35%	55%	90%
Renal elimination	27%	80%	50%	30%
Substrate of CYP3A4	Yes	No	Yes	Yes
Substrate of P-gp	Yes	Yes	Yes	Yes
Dialyzable	No	Yes	No	No

Table 1.
Pharmacological properties of DOACs.

the risk of recurrent VTE. Finally, apixaban, rivaroxaban, and dabigatran have been approved by US FDA and European Medical Agency (EMA) for thrombo-prophylaxis post orthopedic surgeries (i.e., knee and hip replacements). Apixaban and rivaroxaban are approved for post-knee and hip replacement surgeries, and dabigatran is only approved for post-hip replacement surgery. In addition, rivaroxaban is also approved for VTE prophylaxis in acutely ill medical patients at risk for thromboembolic complications, not at high risk of bleeding [9]. **Table 2** illustrates the usual dosing recommendations for the various indications.

3.4 Monitoring

DOACs possess the advantage of having predictable pharmacokinetic and pharmacodynamic properties making their regular monitoring of blood levels or coagulation factors not necessary. This provides a great advantage and more convenience to patients than the traditional anticoagulant warfarin. Currently, there are no validated and clinically feasible tests to measure the anticoagulant effect of DOACs on daily basis. Besides, routine monitoring of kidney function is necessary to ensure appropriate clearance of DOACs as all of them have varying degrees of renal elimination. This becomes of high importance when dealing with end-stage renal disease patients or patients on hemodialysis. Monitoring hepatic function every 6 to 12 months is recommended as all DOACs except dabigatran are metabolized by the liver. Regular follow-up on patient adherence is also encouraged to ensure the safety and efficacy of the anticoagulation given their short duration of action [9].

3.5 Side effects

As with all anticoagulants, the main severe and concerning side effect is bleeding. Careful watching of signs and symptoms of bleeding and proper patient education on identifying them is crucial. Dyspepsia is another reported side effect more linked to dabigatran. Taking dabigatran with food should help with minimizing dyspepsia as the body tolerates the medication with time [10].

3.6 Choosing an anticoagulant agent

Warfarin could be an appealing anticoagulant option in many cases. For example, it could be an adequate option to be sued in patients with an estimated creatinine

Apixaban	Dabigatran	Edoxaban	Rivaroxaban
Stroke prevention in nonvalvular atrial fibrillation (NVAF)			
5 mg PO BID 2.5 mg PO BID if two of the following occurs: • Age ≥ 80 years • Scr ≥ 1.5 mg/dl • Weight ≤ 60 kg	150 mg PO BID	60 mg PO once daily • Not recom-mended with CrCl > 95 ml/min	20 mg PO once daily
Treatment of acute venous thromboembolism (VTE)			
10 mg PO BID for 7 days, then 5 mg PO BID	Following 5-10 days of initial parenteral therapy: 150 mg PO BID	Following 5-10 days of initial parenteral therapy: • Weight > 60 kg: 60 mg PO once daily • Weight ≤ 60 kg: 30 mg PO once daily	15 mg PO BID for 21 days, then 20 mg PO once daily
Reduction in the risk of recurrent VTE			
2.5 mg PO BID	150 mg PO BID	Not approved	10 mg PO once daily
Post-knee/hip replacement DVT prophylaxis			
2.5 mg PO BID 12-24 hours post-op • Hip replacement duration: 35 days • Knee replacement duration: 12 days	Hip replacement only: 110 mg PO 1-4 hours post-surgery, then 220 mg PO once daily for 28-35 days	Not approved	10 mg PO once daily 6-10 hours post-op • Hip replacement duration: 35 days • Knee replacement duration: 12 days
VTE prophylaxis in acutely ill medical patients at risk for thromboembolic complications, not at high risk of bleeding			
Not approved	Not approved	Not approved	10 mg PO once daily in the hospital and after hospital discharge for a total duration of 31-39 days

Table 2.
DOACs approved indications and recommended doses for normal kidney patients.

clearance (CrCl) of less than 30 mL/min as those individuals were excluded from many clinical trials that compared warfarin to the DOACs. Also, it could be used in patients with poor medication adherence. This is mainly because many of the currently available DOACs are dosed to be taken twice daily. This could affect patient adherence. In addition, the presence of laboratory assessment modalities like the INR can identify poor medication adherence. Despite the long list of interacting medications with warfarin, the use of *warfarin could be preferred as dose adjustments based on INR monitoring can facilitate titration of the anticoagulant response. Warfarin remains the least expensive anticoagulant currently available. This could make it a reasonable option for individuals who cannot afford the more costly options* [11].

DOACs are considered the first line option in many indications given their predicted pharmacokinetics and pharmacodynamics which minimizes the need for regular drug monitoring compared to warfarin. They are dosed either once daily or twice daily and do not have significant drug-food interactions. Patients with various degrees of renal impairment (i.e. CrCL <30 ml/min) were excluded from the DOACs' pivotal trials, therefore their use in this certain population is debatable. However, apixaban, for example has good pharmacokinetic data supporting its use in hemodialysis (HD) patients as it has very low renal clearance that accounts for only 25%. Currently, apixaban is recommended for stroke prevention in atrial fibrillation patients with end stage renal disease (ESRD) on HD. On the other hand, patients with poor compliance may benefit more from being on warfarin rather than DOACs as the effect of warfarin stays longer than DOACs. If a patient misses one dose of warfarin, the INR would still be in the therapeutic range for one or more days. Finally, the need to monitor kidney function with DOACs still exists and crucial to assess the need for renal dose adjustments [12, 13].

3.7 Periprocedural management of anticoagulation

Management of anticoagulation before and after surgeries such as thrombectomy is very crucial safety step to ensure safe and effective surgical interventions with minimal chances for bleedings. The appropriate knowledge of anticoagulants pharmacokinetics properties and the degree of bleeding risk of the procedure are two essential factors to formulate an appropriate periprocedural anticoagulation plan. Special considerations should be taken with individuals with impaired renal or liver functions [14].

Procedure Bleeding Risk	DOAC	Warfarin
Minimal	• Omit anticoagulant on the day of procedure	• No interruption needed
Low	• Omit anticoagulant one day before the procedure • Reinitiate anticoagulant one day after the procedure • For individuals receiving dabigatran with CrCl 30 to 50 mL/min: omit two days before procedure.	• Assess thromboembolic risk: • Low – moderate risk: interrupt 5 days before the procedure without parenteral anticoagulant bridging • High risk: interrupt 5 days before the procedure with parenteral anticoagulant bridging
Moderate	• Omit anticoagulant one day before the procedure • Reinitiate anticoagulant one day after the procedure	• Assess thromboembolic risk: • Low – moderate risk: interrupt 5 days before the procedure without parenteral anticoagulant bridging • High risk: interrupt 5 days before the procedure with parenteral anticoagulant bridging • Reinitiate warfarin postoperatively once hemostasis is attained
High	• Omit anticoagulant two day before the procedure • Reinitiate anticoagulant two day after the procedure • For individuals receiving dabigatran with CrCl 30 to 50 mL/min: omit four days before procedure	• interrupt 5 days before the procedure with parenteral anticoagulant bridging • Reinitiate warfarin postoperatively once hemostasis is attained

Table 3.
Periprocedural management of anticoagulants.

In patients who are on a DOAC and going into a minimal risk procedure, omitting one dose of the anticoagulant on the day of the procedure is sufficient. However, in low or moderate risk procedures, the anticoagulant should be omitted for one day before the procedure and restart one day after the procedure. In high-risk procedures, omitting the DOAC agent two days before and after the procedure would reasonable. **Table 3** summarizes the periprocedural management of anticoagulants.

On the other side, patients who are on warfarin and undergoing minimal risk procedures, interruption of anticoagulation is not necessary. However, in other low and moderate risk procedures, warfarin should be interrupted with mostly no need for bridging. In high risk, interruption of anticoagulation is needed with bridging. Discontinuation of warfarin should be done five days before the procedure. When bridging is required, starting enoxaparin three days before the procedure is reasonable with last dose being given 24 hours before the procedure. In patients with various degrees of renal impairments may require longer interruption periods as clearance of the anticoagulant may become delayed. **Table 3** summarizes the periprocedural management of anticoagulants.

4. Reversal Agents

4.1 Warfarin reversal modalities

Holding or discontinuing warfarin as a solo strategy may be adequate in asymptomatic patients with an elevated INR value and a low risk for bleeding. Certain patient may require further agents to be administered such as, Vitamin K (phytonadione), Prothrombin Complex Concentrate (PCC), and Fresh frozen plasma (FFP) [15].

4.1.1 Vitamin K (Phytonadione)

Exogenous vitamin K level helps reestablishing the hepatic formation of vitamin K–dependent clotting factors. When exogenous vitamin K is given, it can continue to be reduced and converted to its active form, KH2, which results with functional clotting factors despite recent warfarin administration. Vitamin K dose and route of administration vary depends on the bleeding magnitude. It can be given as 2–5 mg PO/IV for minor bleeding events and 5–10 IV for major bleed. Although they are rare, anaphylactic reactions and temporary warfarin resistance have been reported with vitamin K use IV vitamin K normalizes the INR quicker than PO. It only takes 8–12 hours with IV administration and might take up to 24–48 hours following oral administration [15].

4.1.2 Prothrombin Complex Concentrate (PCC)

Clotting factor replenishing, and it can enchase platelet activation. These clotting factors are 25-fold more concentrated than blood. Recombinant activated factor VII (FVIIa) (NovoSeven®) contains activated factor VII can directly activate thrombin generation by binding to tissue factor. PCC products are differentiated by the type of clotting factors they consist of. The 3-factor PCC consist of clotting factors II, IX, and X. The 4-factor PCC 4 consist of clotting factors II, IX, X, and VII (4PCC). Activated 4-factor PCC consist of II, IX, X, and VIIa. All PCC products have natural anticoagulants protein C and protein S. and all PCC products contain heparin, except Profilnine® (3-factor PCC) [15].

PCC dosing is based on factor IX and activated versus non-activated pertains to factor VII. Normally each single-dose vial of PCC is mixed with 10–40 mL of sterile water. Fixed dose PCC for non-intracranial hemorrhagic (ICH) bleed is usually 1000 units while in ICH, it is 1500–2000 units. The other modality to dose PCC is INR and weight driven dose. In patients with INR of 2 to less than 4, the dose is 25 units/kg. In patients with INR of 4–6,, the dose is 35 units/kg. In patients with INR of more than 6, the dose is 50 units/kg. PCC dose might need to be rounded up or down to the nearest available vial size. The acceptable dose adjusting margin is institution dependent (usually 5–10%). Infusion related allergic reactions, heparin-induced thrombocytopenia (with exception of Profilnine®) and low acceptable risk of thrombosis have been reported in patients receiving PCC therapy [15].

4.1.3 Fresh frozen plasma (FFP)

FFP is not a specific reversal agent. It contains all coagulation factors, including II, VII, IX, and X in diluted inactive form. Moreover, it contains fibrinogen and platelet. There is no specific recommendation when it comes to FFP dosing, but usually it is given as 10–30 mL/kg (1-unit FFP has a volume of 250 mL). Transfusion reactions, volume overload, infection, and transfusion-related lung injury have been reported in patients receiving FFP therapy [15].

4.2 Direct thrombin inhibitors reversal agents

4.2.1 Idarucizumab

Idarucizumab is a humanized monoclonal antibody fragment that has been developed specifically to reverse the anticoagulation effect of dabigatran [9]. Idarucizumab is indicated for emergent surgery/urgent procedures In life-threatening or uncontrolled bleeding. It is given as a total dose of 5 grams (two separate doses of 2.5 g diluted in 50 mL vials) intravenous infusion over 5 minutes. Idarucizumab carries a warning for inducing thromboembolic events. The thrombotic rate in REVERSE-AD trial was 4.8% at 1 month. The risks of hypersensitivity and severe adverse reactions in patients with hereditary fructose intolerance are reported in the packaging insert due to sorbitol excipient. Among patients who received Idarucizumab, 5% or more experienced hypokalemia, pneumonia, pyrexia, and delirium [9].

4.2.2 Prothrombin Complex Concentrates (PCC)

Inconsistent data was reported regarding the efficacy of PCC in reversing dabigatran based on its laboratory abnormalities. When PCC is used, aPCC such as FEIBA may be preferred. The thrombin generation following PCC administration is dose dependent. Currently most guidelines recommend aPCC 50 units/kg to be given when an emergent reversal is needed for dabigatran. Because of the presence of activated clotting factors, and higher prothrombin and thrombin content in aPCC, the risk of thrombosis is expected to be higher with aPCC than with PCC [9].

4.3 Anti-Xa inhibitors reversal agents

4.3.1 Andexanet alfa

Andexanet alpha is a recombinant modified human "decoy" factor Xa protein, and it works through a competitive binding mechanism with high specificity to direct and indirect anti-Xa agents; to restore the activity of factor Xa and reverses the anticoagulant effect. In May 2018, the FDA approved Andexxa® for the reversal of apixaban and rivaroxaban in the setting of life-threatening or uncontrolled major bleeding. Later, the European Medicine Agency (EMA) gave it a 'conditional authorization' in 2019 using the trade name of (Ondexxya®)[9].

Andexanet alpha dosing is either 400 mg IV bolus followed by continuous IV infusion or 800 mg IV bolus followed by 960 mg continuous IV infusion, based on drug, dose, and timing. Treatment with the high dose would cost $49,500 for the drug alone. It is available as 100-mg dry powder vials. It needs to be reconstituted with 10 mL SWFI with typical dissolution time of 3 minutes. Most common reported issues related to andexanet alfa include flushing and fever which may be an infusion related side effect in study performed in healthy volunteers. Albeit the decoy mechanism of action of this drug, the most common side effects in patients with major bleeding events were thromboembolism including DVTs, myocardial infarction and ischemic stroke which was reported in 10% in the ANEXXA-4 trial.

4.3.2 Prothrombin Complex Concentrates (PCCs)

Variable data have been reported on the role of PCC in anti-Xa as potential reversal strategies. Multiple guidelines suggest using PCCs as alternative method to andexanet alfa. However, multiple reports demonstrated similar efficacy and safety profile for PCCs when used for major bleed induced by rivaroxaban, apixaban, or edoxaban. Many clinicians may prefer PCCs over andexanet alfa based on the cost difference in addition to the lack of high-quality head-to-head comparisons. Dosing may have a range between 25 and 50 units/kg based on actual body weight [9].

5. Ongoing research on anticoagulant therapy

The anti-factor Xa inhibitors have achieved so many milestones and currently are recommended by most well-respected clinical guidelines. This mechanism of action is becoming so appealing for many manufacturers to design new agents that specifically target factor Xa. Darexaban and nokxaban are two new potential agents that may see the light soon and attain the guidelines recommendations for many clinical indications. They have still not been approved by neither the US FDA nor the EMA but their Phase II trials are promising with comparable safety and efficacy data to current approved DOACs. On the other side, currently approved DOACs are being tested for many other indications and we may see further utilization of these agents on a wider range of patient population. Drugs targeting other coagulation factors such as factor XI and XII are also being developed [16–19].

6. Conclusion

Several anticoagulant agents could be used to manage thrombotic events. However, it is essential to consider thrombectomy over anticoagulant therapy in acute settings. This is mainly due to the fact that limited data exist on the use of VKA or DOACs in the acute treatment of patients with ischemic stroke. Anticoagulants could be reserved as a secondary prevention strategy in many thrombotic disorders.

Conflict of interest

The authors declare no conflict of interest.

Notes/thanks/other declarations

None.

Author details

Mohammed Aldhaeefi, Abdulrahman Alshaya, Khalid Bin Saleh, Omar Alshaya
and Hisham Badreldin*
Department of Pharmacy Practice, College of Pharmacy, King Saud bin Abdulaziz
University for Health Sciences, Riyadh, Saudi Arabia

*Address all correspondence to: hishamahmed87@gmail.com

IntechOpen

References

[1] Dahlbäck B. Blood coagulation. Lancet. 2000;355(9215):1627-1632.

[2] Lim GB. Milestone 1: Discovery and purification of heparin. Nat Rev Cardiol. 2017 Dec 14.

[3] Lim GB. Milestone 2: Warfarin: from rat poison to clinical use. Nat Rev Cardiol. 2017 Dec 14.

[4] Cully M. Milestone 9: Ximelagatran sets the stage for NOACs. Nat Rev Cardiol. 2017 Dec 14.

[5] Huynh K. Milestone 10: Era of the NOACs. Nat Rev Cardiol. 2017 Dec 14.

[6] Harter K, Levine M, Henderson SO. Anticoagulation drug therapy: a review. West J Emerg Med. 2015 Jan;16(1):11-17.

[7] Badreldin H, Nichols H, Rimsans J, Carter D. Evaluation of anticoagulation selection for acute venous thromboembolism. J Thromb Thrombolysis. 2017 Jan;43(1):74-78.

[8] Weitz JI. Factor Xa and thrombin as targets for new oral anticoagulants. Thromb Res. 2011 Jan;127 Suppl:S5-12.

[9] Chaudhary R, Sharma T, Garg J, Sukhi A, Bliden K, Tantry U, et al. Direct oral anticoagulants: a review on the current role and scope of reversal agents. J Thromb Thrombolysis. 2020 Feb;49(2):271-286.

[10] Connors JM. Testing and monitoring direct oral anticoagulants. Blood. 2018;132(19):2009-2015.

[11] Wadsworth D, Sullivan E, Jacky T, Sprague T, Feinman H, Kim J. A review of indications and comorbidities in which warfarin may be the preferred oral anticoagulant. J Clin Pharm Ther. 2021 Jun;46(3):560-570.

[12] January CT, Wann LS, Calkins H, Chen LY, Cigarroa JE, Cleveland JC, et al. 2019 AHA/ACC/HRS Focused Update of the 2014 AHA/ACC/HRS Guideline for the Management of Patients With Atrial Fibrillation: A Report of the American College of Cardiology/American Heart Association Task Force on Clinical Practice Guidelines and the Heart R. J Am Coll Cardiol. 2019;74(1):104-132.

[13] Hindricks G, Potpara T, Dagres N, Arbelo E, Bax JJ, Blomström-Lundqvist C, et al. 2020 ESC Guidelines for the diagnosis and management of atrial fibrillation developed in collaboration with the European Association for Cardio-Thoracic Surgery (EACTS): The Task Force for the diagnosis and management of atrial fibrillation of the Europea. Eur Heart J. 2021;42(5):373-498.

[14] Doherty JU, Gluckman TJ, Hucker WJ, Januzzi JL, Ortel TL, Saxonhouse SJ, et al. 2017 ACC Expert Consensus Decision Pathway for Periprocedural Management of Anticoagulation in Patients With Nonvalvular Atrial Fibrillation: A Report of the American College of Cardiology Clinical Expert Consensus Document Task Force. J Am Coll Cardiol. 2017;69(7):871-898.

[15] Makris M, van Veen JJ, Maclean R. Warfarin anticoagulation reversal: management of the asymptomatic and bleeding patient. J Thromb Thrombolysis. 2010 Feb;29(2):171-181.

[16] Iwatsuki Y, Sato T, Moritani Y, Shigenaga T, Suzuki M, Kawasaki T, et al. Biochemical and pharmacological profile of darexaban, an oral direct factor Xa inhibitor. Eur J Pharmacol. 2011 Dec 30;673(1-3):49-55.

[17] Kadokura T, Kashiwa M, Groenendaal D, Heeringa M, Mol R, Verheggen F, et al. Clinical pharmacokinetics, pharmacodynamics,

safety and tolerability of darexaban, an oral direct factor Xa inhibitor, in healthy Caucasian and Japanese subjects. Biopharm Drug Dispos. 2013 Nov;34(8):431-441.

[18] Choi HY, Choi S, Kim YH, Lim HS. Population Pharmacokinetic and Pharmacodynamic Modeling Analysis of GCC-4401C, a Novel Direct Factor Xa Inhibitor, in Healthy Volunteers. CPT pharmacometrics Syst Pharmacol. 2016;5(10):532-543.

[19] Weitz JI, Chan NC. Advances in Antithrombotic Therapy. Arterioscler Thromb Vasc Biol. 2019;39(1):7-12.

Chapter 2

Recent Advances in Thrombolysis and Thrombectomy in Acute Ischemic Stroke Treatment: Neurologist's and Interventional Neuroradiologist's Perspective

Pinar Gelener and Süha Halil Akpinar

Abstract

As stroke is still the leading cause of disability and mortality worldwide, it is promising that there has been a significant change in the acute treatment options for the patients presenting with acute ischemic stroke over the last 23 years after the approval of alteplase. Vascular recanalization of the occluded artery by endovascular methods with or without thrombolysis has shown improved clinical outcomes, particularly after randomized control trials (RCTs), which were conducted between December 2010, and December 2014. These trials will be discussed in more detail the below following sections of this chapter. Successful emergency reperfusion conducted on time still remains the most important determinant of good clinical outcome.

Keywords: thrombectomy, advances, acute ischemic stroke

1. Introduction - Neurologist's perspective

1.1 Choices for intravenous thrombolysis

Vascular recanalization of the occluded artery by endovascular methods with or without thrombolysis has shown improved clinical outcomes, particularly after randomized control trials which were conducted between December 2010, and December 2014. These trials will be discussed in more detail the below following sections of this chapter. Successful emergency reperfusion conducted on time still remains the most important determinant of good clinical outcome [1].

Another choice for rtPA is tenecteplase, which is a variant of rtPA with a longer half-life and greater fibrin specificity. The Norwegian Tenecteplase Stroke Trial 2 (NOR-TEST 2) is still continuing, but the NOR-TEST 1 trial showed that tenecteplase has a similar safety profile to alteplase but it is not superior [2].

According to the Tenecteplase versus Alteplase, before Endovascular Therapy for Ischemic Stroke (EXTEND-IA TNK) trial that included patients with acute proximal intracranial artery occlusion eligible for mechanical thrombectomy, tenecteplase has a higher reperfusion incidence and better functional outcomes when compared to alteplase [3].

1.2 Patients exceeding time-limit: presenting from very-late to unknown "last-seen-well" time

There is a group of patients in the extended time window for whom acute reperfusion therapies may still be effective. Perfusion brain imaging is crucial in this group of patients [4].

1.3 Intravenous rtPA across 4.5–9 hours

A recent meta-analysis of the EXTEND and EPITHET Randomized Clinical Trials revealed that reperfusion with IV alteplase reduced disability in patients with acute ischemic stroke (AIS) within 4.5–9 hours after symptom onset or wake-up onset, who were selected by perfusion imaging mismatch, without increasing the risk of symptomatic intracerebral hemorrhage [5].

The efficacy and safety of MRI-Based Thrombolysis in the Wake-Up Stroke (WAKE-UP) trial including patients beyond 4.5 hours who woke up with a stroke or could not identify the onset and had a diffusion and flair mismatch, also showed receiving IV rtPA was beneficial [6].

The ongoing "Tenecteplase in wake-up ischemic stroke" (TWIST) trial will answer further questions about the superiority of tenecteplase over standard treatments for acute ischemic stroke patients in the extended time window [7].

1.4 Time limit for endovascular therapies

The first two trials DAWN (the DWI or CTP Assessment with clinical mismatch in the triage of wake-up and late presenting strokes undergoing neurointervention) and DEFUSE 3 (Diffusion and Perfusion Imaging Evaluation for Understanding Stroke Evolution 3) showed dramatic benefit with regard to thrombectomy in patients who had been last well within previous 6–24 hours with radiologic criteria indicating a mismatch between ischemic core and penumbra by perfusion or diffusion-weighted images [8, 9].

The aim of the diffusion/perfusion images is to identify the ischemic penumbra which is the salvageable hypoperfused (but not yet infarcted) region [4].

It is known that in patients with AIS due to large vessel occlusion (LVO) who present very late or who's last seen well period unknown, this may persist beyond 16 hours according to baseline ischemic core, collateral situation status, and perfusion parameters. It is also suggested that the target mismatch pattern may persist up to several days after symptom onset in AIS with large vessel occlusion. In another series of patients with anterior LVO who were evaluated 16 hours after onset, one-third of them had salvageable tissues [10–12].

According to a recent study, patients with acute anterior circulation last vessel occlusion presenting beyond 16 hours up to 10 days from the time they were last seen well, in whom the symptoms slowly progressed, benefited from endovascular treatment. According to the protocol of this study, collateral circulation and perfusion images were evaluated and patients were selected based on core-penumbra mismatch. Good collateral circulation was defined as filling 50% or more middle cerebral artery pial arterial circulation in computed tomography (CT) scan or Magnetic Resonance (MR) angiography [10, 13].

1.5 The role of collateral flow

The primary collaterals refer to the circle of Willis whereas secondary refers to ophthalmic and leptomeningeal arteries and tertiary collaterals to newly developed vessels due to angiogenesis [14, 15].

Leptomeningeal collateral circulation develops chronologically by several compensatory metabolic, hemodynamic, and neural responses. This collateral circulation shows great variability in each individual according to age, genetics, anatomical variations, serum glucose level, and metabolic syndrome [10, 16, 17].

Collateral flow plays a very important role in ensuring that the ischemic penumbra remains viable in patients receiving reperfusion therapies consisting of chemical thrombolysis with alteplase and/or mechanical thrombectomy. The presence of collateral blood supply preserves cerebral perfusion and helps the survival of the hypoperfused ischemic penumbra [4, 18].

Collateral circulation is parallel to better clinical outcomes in AIS patients receiving acute reperfusion therapies, as well as in patients with acute intracranial large vessel occlusions and distal arterial occlusions [19, 20].

There are recent advances in neuroimaging in the evaluation of ischemic penumbra and pial collateral vessels. Vessel-encoded multi-post labeling delay arterial spin labeling (ASL) is a non-invasive, non-contrast magnetic resonance imaging (MRI) measuring collateral perfusion and delayed blood arrival in acute stroke patients [21].

1.6 Patients with mild or rapidly improving deficits and low National Institutes of Health Stroke Scale (NIHSS) scores

It is known that the National Institutes of Health Stroke Scale (NIHSS) score is weighted toward anterior circulation strokes and represents posterior circulation stroke symptoms with lower cutoff values [22].

Although the NIHSS is a predictor of overall AIS outcomes, this does not apply to patients with low NIHSS scores. There is significant variability in the outcomes of patients with AIS and low NIHSS scores, which demonstrates the limitation of NIHSS as a screening tool for treatment eligibility [23, 24].

A patient NIHSS score of 5 or less should be assessed with extra care before the decision to administer rtPA, particularly for those presenting with hemianopia. The "Potential of rtPA for Ischemic Strokes with Mild Symptoms" (PRISMS) trial suggested benefits in terms of thrombolysis in patients with minor non-disabling strokes [4, 25].

Patients with AIS and LVO who present with only mild neurological deficits (NIHSS scores equal or lower than 5) who are treated with IV thrombolysis alone are at risk of early neurological deterioration and poor 3-month outcomes. The two independent predictors of this deterioration are more proximal occlusion sites and thrombus length (according to a Youden index of 9 mm or longer). Bridging therapy, IV rtpA followed by endovascular intervention may be reasonable in this high-risk patient group [26, 27].

Two very important ongoing clinical trials are investigating endovascular thrombectomy in patients with acute large vessel occlusion strokes and low NIHSS score ≤ 5: "Endovascular Therapy for Low NIHSS Ischemic Strokes" (ENDOLOW) and "Minor Stroke Therapy Evaluation" (MOSTE) [23].

1.7 Patients on anticoagulant therapies

According to current guidelines, IV rtPA can only be administered to acute ischemic patients on warfarin if the international normalized ratio (INR) is ≤1.7 without increasing the risk of symptomatic intracranial hemorrhage [28]. The situation in patients on direct oral anticoagulant (DOAC) treatment is more complex as there is no available standardized rapid test to measure DOAC activity (complexities). According to American Heart and Stroke Association guidelines, tPA cannot be given as a treatment in AIS patients if DOAC use is suspected within the past 48 hours [1].

Idarucizumab reverses dabigatran rapidly and irreversibly and andexanet aplha reverses most of the DOACs' anticoagulant activity but it needs a continuous infusion. There is still uncertainty surrounding the treatment of this patient group with rtPA after using reversal agents [29, 30].

In patients taking DOAC with proven AIS with large vessel occlusion, direct endovascular thrombectomy without bridging with IV thrombolysis is preferred especially when thrombectomy can be provided without delay [30].

Recent data suggests that selected patients on DOAC therapy have similar bleeding risks after IV rtPA compared to those who are not. Drug-specific coagulation assays like calibrated anti-Xa activity measure DOAC levels to identify patients with low anticoagulant activity. Thromboelastography is a novel tool used for measuring the viscoelastic properties of clotting blood and the safe threshold for thrombolysis [30–33].

1.8 Patient care after reperfusion therapies

Besides the importance of reperfusion therapies, hemodynamic management and early recognition and treatment of brain edema, infections, and cardiac arrhythmias and failure are critical. Collateral flow can be supported by avoiding sudden drops in blood pressure and the administration of intravenous fluids or vasopressors [4].

According to a recent study from Italy involving patients receiving endovascular treatment for acute stroke, general anesthesia during mechanical thrombectomy was associated with worse functional outcomes compared with conscious sedation and local anesthesia, whereas recanalization success rates did not differ [34].

Both hypoglycemia and hyperglycemia should be avoided in patients with acute ischemic stroke. According to the "Stroke Hyperglycemia Insulin Network Effort (SHINE)" randomized trial, intensive treatment of hyperglycemia (with target 80–130 mg/dl) did not improve functional outcome in patients with acute ischemic stroke when compared to standard treatment (with target 80–179 mg/dl) [35].

According to a collaborative pooled analysis of acute ischemic stroke patients treated by thrombectomy; a systolic blood pressure value of 157 mm Hg predicted the lowest all-cause death rate. It should also be kept in mind that baseline high SBP might reflect the autoregulative hemodynamic intracranial mechanism for the need of good collaterals in large vessel occlusion strokes [36, 37].

Although the current American Heart Association/American Stroke Association guidelines recommend SBP <180 mmHg and DBP <105 mmHg during and after mechanical thrombectomy, evidence for optimal management is limited. Among acute stroke patients with large vessel occlusion treated with mechanical thrombectomy, elevated blood pressure is associated with adverse outcomes before, during, and after the procedure [38].

In some trials, in AIS patients within 6 hours of symptom onset, blood pressure was maintained ≤180–105 mm Hg for the first 24 hours after reperfusion therapies whereas systolic blood pressure was recommended to be <140 mmHg for the first 24 hours in patients with complete recanalization [8, 13].

1.9 Recent news

According to a newly conducted trial involving 41 centers in China, endovascular thrombectomy alone was non-inferior on functional outcome compared to IV alteplase administered within 4.5 hours in AIS from LVO in anterior circulation [39].

2. Interventional radiologist's perspective

2.1 Introduction

Thrombus aspiration and Stent Assisted Thrombectomy (SAT) used either in combination or alone are today the most accepted interventional methods in acute ischemic stroke treatment in large vessel occlusions [40, 41].

The efficacy of the endovascular stroke treatment (EVT) is dependent on the time last seen well and the patient's admittance, imaging methods used to decide whether the patient is eligible for stroke treatment, the technique of thrombectomy with or without bridging, the number of passes during stent retrieval and also the clot type.

2.2 Stroke time and patient's admittance

Admittance of stroke patients to stroke centers was initially made according to two methods. These were, "drip and ship"; putting the patient on a thrombolysis drip after excluding the intracranial hemorrhage mostly by non-contrast CT scan at the closest stroke center and then transferring them to an endovascular center where the endovascular stroke treatment (EVT) is performed. On the other hand, the patient can be admitted directly to an endovascular stroke center to receive the EVT from an experienced stroke team, which is referred to as "direct to mother-ship" [42].

Today, alternative methods are suggested for the transportation of stroke patients.

Mobile stroke units consist of an ambulance equipped with a Computed Tomography (CT) scanner so that suspected stroke patients can have their initial noncontrast CT taken to exclude other causes to allow thrombolysis to be started on the way to the endovascular center [43].

The other option is for a mobile stroke team to evaluate the patient's scans and travel to the hospital with appropriate equipment to conduct an EVT without a neuro interventional team. When the decision is made to intervene, the contact hospital prepares the patient at the local hospital according to the clinical and imaging findings and will also call the anesthesiology team to the angio süite, thus reducing the unwanted delays caused by transfers while the neuro interventional team travels to the hospital to perform the EVT [44].

2.3 Imaging methods

Endovascular stroke treatment was applied within 6 hours in the initial RCTs which resulted in the implementation of the EVT according to AHA/ASA guidelines [45]. However, it was subsequently identified that some patients could still have good results with EVT, even after the 6-hour time limit was exceeded. New imaging-based new trials were introduced to identify why some patients still benefit from EVT even after the eligible time period. According to the latest DAWN and DEFUSE 3 trials, which focused on wake-up and late presenting strokes, the role of multimodal imaging has led to EVT being extended to 24 hours [8, 9].

Most centers apply Computed Tomography (CT) based imaging, which as a start noncontrast CT imaging is frequently used to estimate the ischemic core according to the Alberta Stroke Programme Early CT score (ASPECTS) and to exclude the presence of cerebral hemorrhage. This is followed by CT angiography to identify the level of occlusion as well as the anatomical challenges for procedural planning.

Computed tomography perfusion (CTP) and Diffusion weighted imaging (DWI) are used to identify the core, ischemic penumbra, degree of collaterals, and information of occluded vessels. These data obtained from advanced imaging show that the effectiveness of EVT is not only time-dependent, resulting in "Imaging is Brain" concept instead of "Time is Brain", especially at late attended cases. The 2018 AHA/ASA guidelines recommend the inclusion of CTP, DWI, or Perfusion imaging for the standard evaluation of patients admitted within 6–24 hours. According to imaging cerebral blood flow (CBF) below 30% is defined as infarct core and in DEFUSE 3 T-max more than 6 seconds or apparent diffusion coefficient (ADC) image less than 620 Ym^2/s is used to define the penumbra. Patients with a clinical mismatch (mismatch between the size of infarction and the clinical defect) or patients with target perfusion mismatch (mismatch between the size of infarction and the perfusion lesion) concept were used to define the penumbra and calculate with imaging measurements its ratio to core infarction [46]. Multiphase CTP is also used to define the collateral supply at the risked parenchyma as good collaterals have a reduced rate of infarct growth [47, 48].

2.4 The technique of thrombectomy

Thrombus Aspiration and Stent Assisted Thrombectomy (SAT) used either in combination or alone are now the most accepted interventional methods in acute ischemic stroke treatment in large vessel occlusions. Different thrombectomy stent types and large bore aspiration catheters are introduced to increase the efficacy of endovascular stroke treatment and clot retrieval. The method used in endovascular stroke treatment for large vessel occlusions is mostly made according to the vessel involved, for example, the treatment of internal carotid artery (ICA) orifice, cervical or intracranial parts, or T occlusions is preferably started with thrombus aspiration, whereas SAT is usually applied in middle cerebral artery M2 section of anterior cerebral artery occlusions. However, if the individual methods are not successful alone, combining an aspiration catheter with the thrombectomy stent-method can be used to recanalize the occluded vessel in anterior circulation strokes.

Less RCT is performed in posterior circulation strokes as such cases are less frequent. Direct aspiration as the first pass technique (ADAPT) and stent retrievers are used to recanalize the occluded artery. One of the latest studies focusing on the influence of mechanical thrombectomy—ADAPT versus primary stent retriever—on basilar artery occlusion showed a successful reperfusion rate of 79%, favorable outcome rate of (mRS 0–2) 36.8%, and an all-cause 90-day mortality rate of 44.2%. ADAPT showed a higher complete reperfusion rate with a shorter duration of the procedure [49].

The latest studies that combined alteplase with stent-assisted thrombectomy to SAT alone have shown the noninferiority of mechanical thrombectomy on functional independence with less intracerebral hemorrhage in the hours following endovascular stroke treatment [50, 51].

The First pass effect is defined as the removal of the clot in stroke patients at the first thrombectomy attempt. The impact of the first pass effect was studied in the "Analysis of revascularization in ischemic stroke with EmboTrap" (ARISE 2) study, which focused on the speed of revascularization and the extent of tissue reperfusion [52]. The reperfusion obtained on the first pass with thrombolysis in cerebral infarction (TICI) score 2b-3 had a shorter procedure time compared to the group who obtained the same TICI result but with more thrombectomy passes. As a result, the 90-day mRS score 0–2 was better compared to the multiple pass group even though same the TICI scores were obtained [53] (**Figures 1** and **2**).

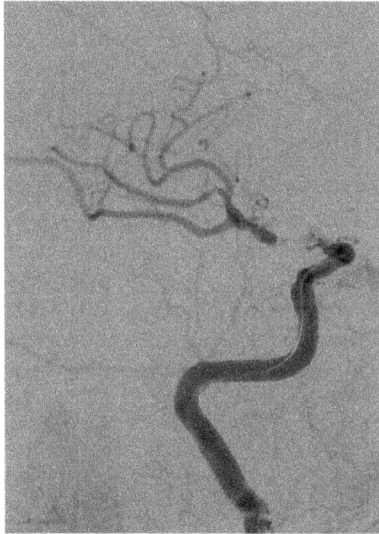

Figure 1.
DSA image of acute right MCA-M1 occlusion and partial recanalization of the occlusion after stent deployment.

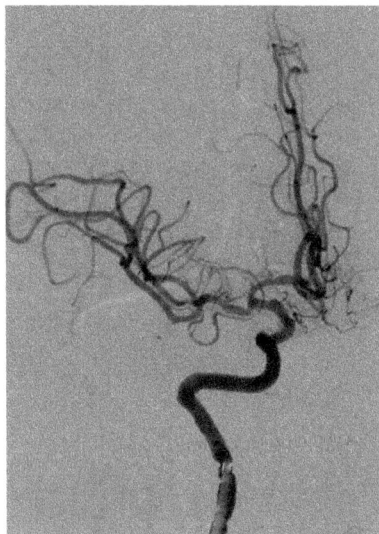

Figure 2.
DSA image after stent assisted thrombectomy with TICI 3 recanalization.

2.5 Clot type

Clot type is also one of the major fields of study in terms of predicting the success of EVT treatment.

It is well known that Erythrocyte-rich thrombi are more responsive to thrombolysis, whereas when the length of the thrombus and its other constituents (i.e., fibrin, platelets, and calcium) result in a reduced success rate of thrombolysis. Although tenecteplase is more fibrin-specific and produces a higher reperfusion rate and better functional outcomes compared to alteplase, its overall success rate is 22% [5, 54, 55].

However, EVT is still less effective in strokes compared to other clot types due to the calcified emboli.

3. Conclusion

The aim of acute ischemic stroke treatment is to reverse the neurologic deficit and to regain function. Successful emergency reperfusion on time with intravenous (iv) thrombolysis with recombinant tissue plasminogen activator (rtPA) and/or endovascular thrombectomy with retrievable stent still remains the most important determinant of good clinical outcome, increasing functionality. Therefore, expanding the availability of reperfusion therapies to all patients including those in the extended period with recommended imaging modalities including collateral flow is crucial (**Table 1**).

I. Patients beyond 4.5-9 hours (receiving IV rtPA)

II. Patients upto 24 hours (receiving endovascular therapies)

III. Patients on warfarin /new oral anticoagulant therapies

IV. Patients with mild deficist and low NIHSS scores

V. Patients with unknown "last seen well"

Table 1.
Acute ischemic stroke patients beyond current guidelines discussed in this chapter.

Conflict of interest

The authors declare no conflict of interest.

Author details

Pinar Gelener[1*] and Süha Halil Akpinar[2]

1 University of Kyrenia, Faculty of Medicine, Department of Neurology, Kyrenia, Cyprus

2 Near East University, Faculty of Medicine, Department of Radiology, Nicosia, Cyprus

*Address all correspondence to: pinar.gelener@kyrenia.edu.tr

IntechOpen

References

[1] Powers WJ, Rabinstein AA, Ackerson T, Adeoye OM, Bambakidis NC, Becker K, et al. Guidelines for the early management of patients with acute ischemic stroke: 2019 update to the 2018 guidelines for the early management of acute ischemic stroke: A guideline for healthcare professionals from the American Heart Association/American Stroke Association. Stroke. 2019;50(12): e344-e418. DOI: 10.1161/STR. 0000000000000211

[2] Logallo N, Kvistad CE, Nacu A, Naess H, Waje-Andreassen U, Asmuss J, et al. The Norwegian tenecteplase stroke trial (NOR-TEST): Randomised controlled trial of tenecteplase vs. alteplase in acute ischaemic stroke. BMC Neurology. 2014;14(1):1-7. DOI: 10.1186/1471-2377-14-106

[3] Campbell BC, Mitchell PJ, Churilov L, et al. Tenecteplase versus alteplase before endovascular thrombectomy (EXTEND-IA TNK): A multicenter, randomized, controlled study. International Journal of Stroke. 2018;13(3):328-334. DOI: 10.1177/ 1747493017733935

[4] Rabinstein AA. Update on treatment of acute ischemic stroke. CONTINUUM: Lifelong Learning in Neurology. 2020;26(2):268-286. DOI: 10.1212/ CON.0000000000000840

[5] Campbell BC, Ma H, Parsons MW, Churilov L, Yassi N, Kleinig TJ, et al. Association of reperfusion after thrombolysis with clinical outcome across the 4.5-to 9-hours and wake-up stroke time window: A meta-analysis of the EXTEND and EPITHET randomized clinical trials. JAMA Neurology. 2021;78(2):236-240. DOI: 10.1001/ jamaneurol.2020.4123

[6] Thomalla G, Boutitie F, Fiebach JB, Simonsen CZ, Nighoghossian N, Pedraza S, et al. Stroke with unknown time of symptom onset: Baseline clinical and magnetic resonance imaging data of the first thousand patients in WAKE-UP (efficacy and safety of MRI-based thrombolysis in wake-up stroke: A randomized, doubleblind, placebo-controlled trial). Stroke. 2017;48(3):770-773. DOI: 10.1161/ STROKEAHA.116.015233

[7] Roaldsen MB, Lindekleiv H, Eltoft A, Jusufovic M, Søyland MH, Petersson J, et al. Tenecteplase in wake-up ischemic stroke trial: Protocol for a randomized-controlled trial. International Journal of Stroke. 14 Jan 2021. pp. 1-5. DOI: 10.1177/1747493020984073

[8] Nogueira RG, Jadhav AP, Haussen DC, Bonafe A, Budzik RF, Bhuva P, et al. Thrombectomy 6 to 24 hours after stroke with a mismatch between deficit and infarct. The New England Journal of Medicine. 2018;378(1):11-21. DOI: 10.1056/NEJMoa1706442

[9] Albers GW, Marks MP, Kemp S, Christensen S, Tsai JP, Ortega-Gutierrez S, et al. Thrombectomy for stroke at 6 to 16 hours with selection by perfusion imaging. The New England Journal of Medicine. 2018;378(8):708-718. DOI: 10.1056/NEJMoa1713973

[10] Kim BJ, Menon BK, Kim JY, Shin DW, Baik SH, Jung C, et al. Endovascular treatment after stroke due to large vessel occlusion for patients presenting very late from time last known well. JAMA Neurology. 2021;78(1):21-29. DOI: 10.1001/ jamaneurol.2020.2804

[11] Christensen S, Mlynash M, Kemp S, Yennu A, Heit JJ, Marks MP, et al. Persistent target mismatch profile > 24 hours after stroke onset in DEFUSE 3. Stroke. 2019;50(3):754-757. DOI: 10.1161/STROKEAHA.118.023392

[12] Rocha M, Desai SM, Jadhav AP, Jovin TG. Prevalence and temporal distribution of fast and slow progressors of infarct growth in large vessel occlusion stroke. Stroke. 2019;**50**(8):2238-2240. DOI: 10.1161/STROKEAHA.118.024035

[13] Goyal M, Demchuk AM, Menon BK, Eesa M, Rempel JL, Thornton J, et al. Randomized assessment of rapid endovascular treatment of ischemic stroke. The New England Journal of Medicine. 2015;**372**(11):1019-1030. DOI: 10.1056/NEJMoa1414905

[14] Liebeskind DS. Collateral circulation. Stroke. 2003;**34**(9): 2279-2284. DOI: 10.1161/01. STR.0000086465.41263.06

[15] Liebeskind DS. The currency of collateral circulation in acute ischemic stroke. Nature Reviews. Neurology. 2009;**5**(12):645-646. DOI: 10.1038/nrneurol.2009.193

[16] Menon BK, Smith EE, Coutts SB, Welsh DG, Faber JE, Goyal M, et al. Leptomeningeal collaterals are associated with modifiable metabolic risk factors. Annals of Neurology. 2013;**74**(2):241-248. DOI: 10.1002/ana.23906

[17] Kao YC, Oyarzabal EA, Zhang H, Faber JE, Shih YY. Role of genetic variation in collateral circulation in the evolution of acute stroke: A multimodal magnetic resonance imaging study. Stroke. 2017;**48**(3):754-761. DOI: 10.1161/STROKEAHA.116.015878

[18] Silva GS, Nogueira RG. Endovascular treatment of acute ischemic stroke. CONTINUUM: Lifelong Learning in Neurology. 2020;**26**(2):310-331. DOI: 10.1212/CON.0000000000000852

[19] Bang OY, Saver JL, Kim SJ, Kim GM, Chung CS, Ovbiagele B, et al. Collateral flow predicts response to endovascular therapy for acute ischemic stroke. Stroke. 2011;**42**(3):693-699. DOI: 10.1161/STROKEAHA.110.595256

[20] Lima FO, Furie KL, Silva GS, Lev MH, Camargo ÉC, Singhal AB, et al. The pattern of leptomeningeal collaterals on CT angiography is a strong predictor of long-term functional outcome in stroke patients with large vessel intracranial occlusion. Stroke. 2010;**41**(10):2316-2322. DOI: 10.1161/STROKEAHA.110.592303

[21] Okell TW, Harston GW, Chappell MA, Sheerin F, Kennedy J, Jezzard P. Measurement of collateral perfusion in acute stroke: A vessel-encoded arterial spin labeling study. Scientific Reports 2019;**9**(1):1-0. DOI:10.1038/s41598-019-44417-7

[22] Sato S, Toyoda K, Uehara T, Toratani N, Yokota C, Moriwaki H, et al. Baseline NIH Stroke Scale Score predicting outcome in anterior and posterior circulation strokes. Neurology. 2008;**70**(24 Part 2):2371-2377. DOI: 10.1212/01.wnl.0000304346.14354.0b

[23] McCarthy DJ, Tonetti DA, Stone J, Starke RM, Narayanan S, Lang MJ, et al. More expansive horizons: A review of endovascular therapy for patients with low NIHSS scores. Journal of NeuroInterventional Surgery. 2021;**13**(2):146-151. DOI: 10.1136/neurintsurg-2020-016583

[24] Kenmuir CL, Hammer M, Jovin T, Reddy V, Wechsler L, Jadhav A. Predictors of outcome in patients presenting with acute ischemic stroke and mild stroke scale scores. Journal of Stroke and Cerebrovascular Diseases. 2015;**24**(7):1685-1689. DOI: 10.1016/j.jstrokecerebrovasdis.2015.03.042

[25] Khatri P, Kleindorfer DO, Devlin T, Sawyer RN, Starr M, Mejilla J, et al. Effect of alteplase vs aspirin on functional outcome for patients with acute ischemic stroke and minor

nondisabling neurologic deficits: The PRISMS randomized clinical trial. Journal of the American Medical Association. 2018;**320**(2):156-166. DOI: 10.1001/jama.2018.8496

[26] Seners P, Hassen WB, Lapergue B, Arquizan C, Heldner MR, Henon H, et al. Prediction of early neurological deterioration in individuals with minor stroke and large vessel occlusion intended for intravenous thrombolysis alone. JAMA Neurology. 2021;**78**(3):321-328. DOI: 10.1001/jamaneurol.2020.4557

[27] Heldner MR, Chaloulos-Iakovidis P, Panos L, Volbers B, Kaesmacher J, Dobrocky T, et al. Outcome of patients with large vessel occlusion in the anterior circulation and low NIHSS score. Journal of Neurology. 2020. pp. 1-12. DOI: 10.1007/s00415-020-09744-0

[28] Mowla A, Memon A, Razavi SM, Lail NS, Vaughn CB, Mohammadi P, et al. Safety of intravenous thrombolysis for acute ischemic stroke in patients taking warfarin with subtherapeutic INR. Journal of Stroke and Cerebrovascular Diseases. 2021;**30**(5):105678. DOI: 10.1016/j.jstrokecerebrovasdis.2021.105678

[29] Czap AL, Grotta JC. Complexities of reperfusion therapy in patients with ischemic stroke pretreated with direct oral anticoagulants: To treat or not, and how? JAMA Neurology. 2021;**78**(5): 517-518. DOI: 10.1001/jamaneurol. 2021.0290

[30] Seiffge DJ, Wilson D, Wu TY. Administering thrombolysis for acute ischemic stroke in patients taking direct oral anticoagulants: To treat or how to treat. JAMA Neurology. 2021;**78**(5):515-516. DOI: 10.1001/jamaneurol. 2021.0287

[31] Macha K, Marsch A, Siedler G, Breuer L, Strasser EF, Engelhorn T, et al. Cerebral ischemia in patients on direct oral anticoagulants: Plasma levels are associated with stroke severity. Stroke.

2019;**50**(4):873-879. DOI: 10.1161/STROKEAHA.118.023877

[32] Seiffge DJ, Traenka C, Polymeris AA, Thilemann S, Wagner B, Hert L, et al. Intravenous thrombolysis in patients with stroke taking rivaroxaban using drug specific plasma levels: Experience with a standard operation procedure in clinical practice. Journal of Stroke. 2017;**19**(3):347. DOI: 10.5853/jos.2017.00395

[33] Bliden KP, Chaudhary R, Mohammed N, Muresan AA, Lopez-Espina CG, Cohen E, et al. Determination of non-vitamin K oral anticoagulant (NOAC) effects using a new-generation thrombelastography TEG 6s system. Journal of Thrombosis and Thrombolysis. 2017;**43**(4):437. DOI: 10.1007/s11239-017-1477-1

[34] Cappellari M, Pracucci G, Forlivesi S, Saia V, Nappini S, Nencini P, et al. General anesthesia versus conscious sedation and local anesthesia during thrombectomy for acute ischemic stroke. Stroke. 2020;**51**(7):2036-2044. DOI: 10.1161/STROKEAHA.120.028963

[35] Bruno A, Durkalski VL, Hall CE, Juneja R, Barsan WG, Janis S, et al. The stroke hyperglycemia insulin network effort (SHINE) trial protocol: A randomized, blinded, efficacy trial of standard vs. intensive hyperglycemia management in acute stroke. International Journal of Stroke. 2014;**9**(2):246-251. DOI: 10.1111/ijs.12045

[36] Maïer B, Gory B, Taylor G, Labreuche J, Blanc R, Obadia M, et al. Mortality and disability according to baseline blood pressure in acute ischemic stroke patients treated by thrombectomy: A collaborative pooled analysis. Journal of the American Heart Association. 2017;**6**(10):e006484. DOI: 10.1161/JAHA.117.006484

[37] Rusanen H, Saarinen JT, Sillanpää N. The association of blood pressure and collateral circulation in hyperacute ischemic stroke patients treated with intravenous thrombolysis. Cerebrovascular Diseases. 2015; **39**(2):130-137. DOI: 10.1159/000371339

[38] Malhotra K, Goyal N, Katsanos AH, Filippatou A, Mistry EA, Khatri P, et al. Association of blood pressure with outcomes in acute stroke thrombectomy. Hypertension. 2020;**75**(3):730-739. DOI: 10.1161/HYPERTENSIONAHA.119.14230

[39] Yang P, Zhang Y, Zhang L, Zhang Y, Treurniet KM, Chen W, et al. Endovascular thrombectomy with or without intravenous alteplase in acute stroke. The New England Journal of Medicine. 2020;**382**(21):1981-1993. DOI: 10.1056/NEJMoa2001123

[40] Castaño C, Dorado L, Guerrero C, Millán M, Gomis M, Perez de la Ossa N, et al. Mechanical thrombectomy with the Solitaire AB device in large artery occlusions of the anterior circulation: A pilot study. Stroke. 2010;**41**:1836-1840. DOI: 10.1161/STROKEAHA.110. 584904

[41] Nayak S, Ladurner G, Killer M. Treatment of acute middle cerebral artery occlusion with a Solitaire AB stent: Preliminary experience. The British Journal of Radiology. 2010;**83**(996):1017-1022. DOI: 10.1259/bjr/42972759

[42] Holodinsky JK, Williamson TS, Kamal N, Mayank D, Hill MD, Goyal M. Drip and ship versus direct to comprehensive stroke center: Conditional probability modeling. Stroke. 2017;**48**(1):233-238. DOI: 10.1161/STROKEAHA.116.014306

[43] Calderon VJ, Kasturiarachi BM, Lin E, Bansal V, Zaidat OO. Review of the mobile stroke unit experience worldwide. Interventional Neurology. 2018;7(6):347-358. DOI: 10.1159/000487334

[44] Wei D, Oxley TJ, Nistal DA, Mascitelli JR, Wilson N, Stein L, et al. Mobile interventional stroke teams lead to faster treatment times for thrombectomy in large vessel occlusion. Stroke. 2017;**48**(12):3295-3300. DOI: 10.1161/STROKEAHA.117.018149

[45] Powers WJ, Derdeyn CP, Biller J, Coffey CS, Hoh BL, Jauch EC, et al. American Heart Association/American Stroke Association focused update of the 2013 guidelines for the early management of patients with acute ischemic stroke regarding endovascular treatment: A guideline for healthcare professionals from the American Heart Association/American Stroke Association. Stroke. 2015;**46**(10): 3020-3035. DOI: 10.1161/ STR.0000000000000074

[46] Albers GW, Lansberg MG, Brown S, Jadhav AP, Haussen DC, Martins SO, et al. Assessment of optimal patient selection for endovascular thrombectomy beyond 6 hours after symptom onset: A pooled analysis of the AURORA database. JAMA Neurology. 2021;**78**(9):1064-1071. DOI: 10.1001/ jamaneurol.2021.2319

[47] García-Tornel A, Carvalho V, Boned S, Flores A, Rodríguez-Luna D, Pagola J, et al. Improving the evaluation of collateral circulation by multiphase computed tomography angiography in acute stroke patients treated with endovascular reperfusion therapies. Interventional Neurology. 2016;**5**(3-4):209-217. DOI: 10.1159/000448525

[48] Piedade GS, Schirmer CM, Goren O, Zhang H, Aghajanian A, Faber JE, et al. Cerebral collateral circulation: A review in the context of ischemic stroke and mechanical thrombectomy. World Neurosurgery. 2019;**122**:33-42. DOI: 10.1016/j.wneu.2018.10.066

[49] Gory B, Mazighi M, Blanc R, Labreuche J, Piotin M, Turjman F, et al.

Mechanical thrombectomy in basilar artery occlusion: Influence of reperfusion on clinical outcome and impact of the first-line strategy (ADAPT vs stent retriever). Journal of Neurosurgery. 2018;**129**(6):1482-1491. DOI: 10.3171/2017.7.JNS171043

[50] Suzuki K, Matsumaru Y, Takeuchi M, Morimoto M, Kanazawa R, Takayama Y, et al. Effect of mechanical thrombectomy without vs with intravenous thrombolysis on functional outcome among patients with acute ischemic stroke: The SKIP randomized clinical trial. Journal of the American Medical Association. 2021;**325**(3):244-253

[51] Jian Y, Zhao L, Jia B, Tong X, Li T, Wu Y, et al. Direct versus bridging mechanical thrombectomy in elderly patients with acute large vessel occlusion: A multicenter cohort study. Clinical Interventions in Aging. 2021;**16**:1265. DOI: 10.1001/jama.2020.23522

[52] Zaidat OO, Bozorgchami H, Ribó M, Saver JL, Mattle HP, Chapot R, et al. Primary results of the multicenter ARISE II study (analysis of revascularization in ischemic stroke with EmboTrap). Stroke. 2018;**49**(5):107-1115. DOI: 10.1161/STROKEAHA.117.020125

[53] Yoo AJ, Andersson T, Ribo M, Bozorgchami H, Liebeskind D, Jadhav A, et al. Abstract TP41: The importance of first pass substantial reperfusion in the ARISE II study. Stroke. 2019;**50**(Suppl_1):ATP41

[54] Campbell BC, Mitchell PJ, Churilov L, Yassi N, Kleinig TJ, Dowling RJ, et al. Tenecteplase versus alteplase before thrombectomy for ischemic stroke. The New England Journal of Medicine. 2018;**378**(17): 1573-1582. DOI: 10.1056/NEJMoa1716405

[55] Dobrocky T, Piechowiak E, Cianfoni A, Zibold F, Roccatagliata L, Mosimann P, et al. Thrombectomy of calcified emboli in stroke. Does histology of thrombi influence the effectiveness of thrombectomy? Journal of NeuroInterventional Surgery. 2018;**10**(4):345-350. DOI: 10.1136/neurintsurg-2017-013226

Chapter 3

Endovascular Treatment for Acute Mesenteric Ischemia

Mu-Yang Hsieh

Abstract

The current standard care for acute mesenteric ischemia involves urgent revascularization and resection of the necrotic bowel. A dedicated protocol for early treatment and urgent revascularization is pivotal to improving diagnostic rate and patient survival. In this chapter, the critical components of diagnosis and treatment protocol are reviewed. Different treatment choices with endovascular approaches are discussed. After endovascular revascularization, a dedicated team consisting of surgeons and critical care specialists are needed to provide post-intervention care and second-look laparoscopy when necessary. In geographic regions where healthcare resources are lacking, a time-efficient strategy adopted by interventional radiologists or cardiologists should be considered to improve patient survival.

Keywords: acute, mesenteric ischemia, endovascular

1. Introduction

1.1 How we begin our treatment protocol

On August 24, 2012, we started our first endovascular treatment for acute mesenteric ischemia. The patient received diagnosis of acute abdomen in the emergent department, and our general surgeon per- formed laparotomy, which found diffuse mesenteric necrosis. After emergent operation, the interven- tional cardiology team was consulted. Endovascular revascularization was performed by Dr. Mu-Yang Hsieh and Dr. Kuei-Chien Tsai. A coronary bare-metal stent was placed to revascularize SMA (superior mesenteric artery) (Integrity, bare-metal stent, 4.0 x 28 mm, Medtronics) (**Figure 1**).

On August 17, 2012, Dr. Mu-Yang Hsieh initiated a draft for Acute Mesenteric Ischemia Protocol. Be- tween 2013 and 2014, interventional radiologist Dr. Chih-Hon Wu provided valuable revision sugges- tions. In the following years, another seven patients received emergent endocvascular revascularization for acute mesenteric ischemia.

1.1.1 The goal of the protocol

1. Initial goals: a definitive invasive angiography become a reasonable options for dignosis improvement. To have an in-hospital monitor program.

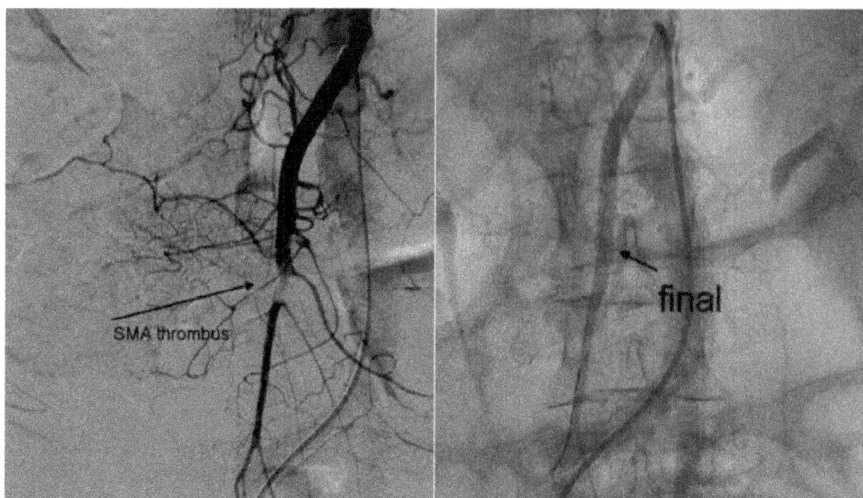

Figure 1.
The angiography found acute superior mesenteric artery occlusion. The flow was re-established after thrombosuction, balloon angioplasty, and stenting with a bare-metal balloon expandable stent (case 1).

2. Intermediate goals: become a center for emergent treatment for acute mesenteric ischemia.

3. Longterm goals: to achieve better survival as reported from previous literatures. Make our one-year survival rate approximate 88%.

1.2 Statistics in our hospital

"Patients only have hours before irreversible gut ischemia ensues, followed by profound distributive shock, and death. (quoted from Moore and Ahn, Chapter 35)."

Bowel ischemia was diagnosed in around 0.1% of hospitalized patients [1]. But the mortality of acute mesenteric ischemia is quite high. In our hospital, about 95%mesenteric ischemia presented with acute abdomen.

Because the diagnosis of acute ischemic bowel is often difficult, we initiated a dedicated diagnosis pro- tocol to improve the patient outcomes. (**Figure 2**):

1. Emergent primary surgery with f/u angio: 4 patients, all received angio, with 2 SMA lesions fixed, survival 75% (3/4).

2. Emergent primary endovascular approach (with second look laparoscopy when indicated): 18 pa- tients, 5 failure, survival 0% (0/5), 13 success, survival 92.3% (12/13), 4 required laparoscopy/laparotomy.

3. Totally conservative management: 6 patients, survival 0% (0/6).

A filling defect (clot) was found in the SMA (**Figure 3**):

1. Early invasive endovascular approach: 8 patients, survival 75% (6/8).

2. Conservative medical management: 5 patients, survival 0% (0/5).

Registry- 2012 to 2020

Registry 2012-2020, N = 28 Focusing on initial strategy	Survival at 7-day
Emergent primary surgery with f/u angio	4 patients, all received angio, with 2 SMA lesions fixed, survival 75% (3/4).
Emergent primary endovascular approach (with second look laparoscopy when indicated)	18 patients, 5 failure, survival 0% (0/5), 13 success, survival 92.3% (12/13), 4 required laparoscopy/laparotomy.
Totally conservative management	6 patients, survival 0% (0/6).

Figure 2.
Our registry 2012–2020, 28 patients in the registry. Survival is categorized by treatment modalities.

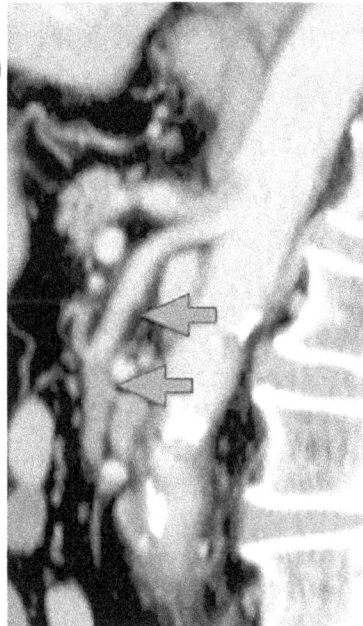

Registry- 2012 to 2020

Focusing on CT findings- filling defect in the SMA	Survival at 7-day
Early invasive endovascular approach	8 patients, survival 75% (6/8).
Conservative medical management	5 patients, survival 0% (0/5).

Figure 3.
The survival categoried by treatment methods after finding clot in the SMA.

2. Literature review

2.1 Review articles and guideline update

Since 2016, there are numerous literature reported that endovascular is better than open surgery [2, 3].

In 2017, a guideline suggested for patients with acute mesenteric ischemia, emergent surgical or endovascular intervention is reasonable.6.

In the absence of RCTs, evidence is based on prospective registries. In the case of embolic occlusion, open and endovascular revascularizations seem to do equally well, whereas, with thrombotic occlusion, endovascular therapy is associated with lower mortality and bowel resection rates. The principles of damage control surgery are important to follow when treating these frail patients. This concept focuses on saving life by restoring normal physiology as quickly as possible, thus avoiding unnecessary time-consuming procedures. Although laparotomy is not mandatory after endovascular therapy in these patients with acute bowel ischaemia, it is often necessary to inspect the bowel. In this setting, second-look laparotomy is also indicated after open revascularization. Intra-arterial catheter thrombolysis of the superior mesenteric artery has been reported with good results. Severe bleeding complications were uncommon, except when intestinal mucosal gangrene was present [4]. See **Figures 3–5**.

2.2 Incidence

Acute mesenteric ischemia is one etiology among many causes of acute abdominal pain (< 1/1000) [5].

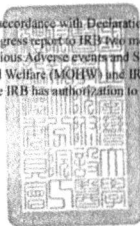

Figure 4.
The internal research board certification.

Recommendations	Class[a]	Level[b]
Diagnosis		
In patients with suspected acute mesenteric ischaemia, urgent CTA is recommended.[179]	I	C
In patients with suspicion of acute mesenteric ischaemia, the measurement of D-dimer should be considered to rule out the diagnosis.[177–179]	IIa	B
Treatment		
In patients with acute thrombotic occlusion of the superior mesenteric artery, endovascular therapy should be considered as first-line therapy for revascularization.[182,184,187,188]	IIa	B
In patients with acute embolic occlusion of the superior mesenteric artery, both endovascular and open surgery therapy should be considered.[182,184,187,188]	IIa	B

Figure 5.
Guideline update in 2017 [4].

2.3 Mortality

In reported literatures, the mortality is around 60–80% among patients with acute mesenteric ischemia [5–8].

2.4 Types of acute mesenteric ischemia

- embolism

- thrombosis

- non-occlusive mesenteric ischemia

- venous thrombosis

Current report addresses that non-occlusive mesenteric ischemia will lead to a worse prognosis.

2.5 Endovascular treatment- cost-effective study

2.5.1 Endovascular interventions decrease the length of hospitalization and are cost-effective in acute mesenteric ischemia

Dr. Erben reported in 2018 that endovascular revascularization for acute mesenteric ischemia is cost-saving, with a lower rate of in-hospital mortality [9].

2.5.2 Endovascular treatment for acute thromboembolic occlusion of the superior Mesen-teric artery and the outcome comparison between endovascular and open Surgi-cal treatments: A retrospective study

Similar good endovascular treatment results were also obtained in a cohort of Chinese population. A table comparing endovascular versus open surgery groups offer a good perspective on this topic (**Table 1**) [10].

2.6 Contemporary management of acute mesenteric ischemia in the Endovascular era

Dr. Lim et al. reported in 2019 that for acute mesenteric ischemia, both open surgery and endovascular revascularization are viable options in the modern era [11]. See: **Tables 2** and **3**.

Variable	Endovascular group (n = 18)	Open surgery group (n = 12)	p	t
Symptom onset to treatment (h)	20.8 ± 15.2	25.8 ± 11.3	0.35	−0.96
Laparotomy required (%/n)	33.33 (6)	58.33 (7)	0.26	
Time to laparotomy (h)	26.3 ± 16.8	18.0 ± 7.7	0.26	1.18
Bowel resection (cm)	88 ± 44	253 ± 103	0.01	3.85
Thirty-day mortality (%/n)	16.7 (3)	33.3 (4)	0.68	

Abbreviations: CA, celiac artery; CT; computed tomography; IMA, inferior mesenteric artery; MI, myocardial infarction; SMA, superior mesenteric artery.
Source: From Kirkpatrick ID, et al.: Biphasic CT with mesenteric CT angiography in the evaluation of acute mesenteric ischemia: initial experience. Radiology. 2003; 229(1):9 l-98.

Table 1.
Therapeutic efficacy between endovascular and open surgery groups [10].

Findings	Acute MI, n = 26	Control, n = 36	Sensitivity (%)	Specificity (%)
Pneumatosis intestinalis	11	0	42	100
SMA or combined CA and IMA occlusion	5	0	19	100
Arterial embolism	3	0	12	100
SMA or portal venous gas	3	0	12	100
Focal lack of bowel wall enhancement	11	1	42	97
Free intraperitoneal air	5	2	19	94
SMA or portal venous thrombosis	4	2	15	94
Solid organ infarction	4	2	15	94
Bowel obstruction	3	2	12	94
Bowel dilatation	17	6	65	93
Mucosal enhancement	12	7	46	81
Bowel wall thickening	22	10	85	72
Mesenteric stranding	23	14	88	61
Ascites	19	24	73	33

Abbreviations: CA, celiac artery; CT; computed tomography; IMA, inferior mesenteric artery; MI, myocardial infarction; SMA, superior mesenteric artery.
Source: From Kirkpatrick ID, et al.: Biphasic CT with mesenteric CT angiography in the evaluation of acute mesenteric ischemia: initial experience. Radiology. 2003; 229 (1):9 l-98.

Table 2.
Important CT image findings for acute mesenteric ischemia [11].

Author (Year)	Data Source	Morbidity	Mortality
Schermerhorn et al. (2009)	Nationwide Inpatient Sample	Length of stay: 9 days vs. 14 days	In-hospital: 16% vs. 39%
		Bowel resection: 28% vs. 37%	
		Acute kidney injury: 11.4% vs. 18.4%	
		Cardiac complication: 2.1% vs. 7.2%	
		Respiratory complication: 1.1% vs. 5.7%	
Block et al. (2010)	Swedish Vascular Registry	Laparotomy: 55% vs. 100%	30-day: 28% vs. 42%
		Bowel resection: 19% vs. 63%	
		Second-look operation: 31% vs. 67%	1 year: 39% vs. 58%
		Short bowel syndrome: 27% vs. 55%	
Arthur et al. (2011)	Single-Center Chart Review	Laparotomy: 69% vs. 100%	36% vs. 50%
		Bowel resection: 52 cm vs. 160 cm	
Beaulieu et al. (2014)	Nationwide Inpatient Sample	Length of stay: 12.9 vs. 17.1 days	In-hospital: 24.9% vs. 39.3%
		Bowel resection: 14.4% vs. 33.4%	
		TPN support: 13.7% vs. 24.4%	
Branco et al. (2015)	Nasional Surgical Quality Improvement Program	Transfusion: 3.7% vs. 19.3%	Odds ratio 0.4 (CI 0.2–0.9)
		Pneumonia: 22.2% vs. 27.8%	
		Sepsis: 25.9% vs. 35.5%	
Arya et al. (2016)	Single-Center Chart Review	Bowel resection: 36.4% vs. 43.5%	30-day: 45.4% vs. 34.8%
		Sepsis: 45.4% vs. 22.7%	
		Re-exploration: 63.6% vs. 56.5%	
		Major morbidity: 63.6% vs. 69.6%	

Abbreviations: CI, confidence interval; TPN, total parenteral nutrition.

Table 3.
Summary of recent literatures (results are endovascular versus open revascularization, respectively) [11].

2.7 Clinical problems

- For the suspected case of acute mesenteric ischemia, is following serum lactate level useful to confirm acute mesenteric ischemia?

  It is not helpful to wait for evidence of increasing serum lactate levels to proceed with further testing; ideally, in fact, intervention would occur in patients with acute mesenteric ischemia before lactic acidosis develops, with the goal of saving additional intestine from full-thickness injury [5].

- When the clinical suspicion of acute mesenteric ischemia is high, we should proceed with CT angiography. And in cases with equivocal CT findings, invasive angiography should be considered.

- In the early phase of abdominal pain, is serum amylase or lipase diagnostic? In the first eight patients of our case series, amylase and lipase is not useful.

• In the first CT study, for patients with no bowel necrosis but still have equivocal CT findings of acute mesenteric ischemia, the best diagnostic method is invasive angiography.

2.8 Primary stenting for acute mesenteric ischemia

Only a few report focused on primary stenting for acute mesenteric ischemia. Dr. Forbrig reported in 2017 with a case series of 19 consecutive patients and demonstrated that endovascular revascularization has high clinical success rates [12].

2.9 Methodology: using Stentriever

Besides balloon angioplasty and stenting, for large thrombus burden, Dr. Miura reported in 2017 that using a stent retriever achieved rapid and good revascularization in a patient with SMA embolism [13].

2.10 Filter protection

Dr. Mendes reported in 2018 that using a distal protection device can redude the event of distal em- bolization [14].

2.11 Special scenario: bypass and its post-OP course

Dr. Morbi reported a patient with acute mesenteric ischemia and the patient received emergent by-pass surgery utilizing an aorto-SMA bypass, with good-quality long saphenous vein and segmental small bowel resection [15].

2.12 Special scenario: dissection

SMA (superior mesenteric artery) dissection has been reported extensively, and the most common problem is when performing open surgery, it is difficult to perform re-entry into the true lumen. The resolution is retrograde open mesenteric stenting (ROMS). The ROMS is performed by opening distal SMA true lumen with placement of a sheath, then proceeding with retrograde wiring and stenting [16].

2.12.1 Classification- SMA dissection

The proposed classification of SMA dissection (**Figure 6**).
For SMA dissection, Dr. Loeffler reported in 2017, that if there was no evidence of bowel necrosis, even in symptomatic SMA dissection, regular medical treatment with follow-up may avoid the necessity of open surgery or endovascular stenting [17].

2.12.2 Endovascular treatment of spontaneous dissections of the superior mesenteric artery

Gobble et al. reported in 2009, included 9 patients (all isolated spontaneous SMA dissection). The treatment modality was variable, including expectant management (4 patients), anticoagulation (2 patients), and endovascular stent placement (3 patients). Among patients who received stenting, acute luminal gain is better [16].
Conservative management of symptomatic spontaneous isolated dissection of the superior mesenteric artery has been reported to be successful. **Cho2009**

Morphological Classification

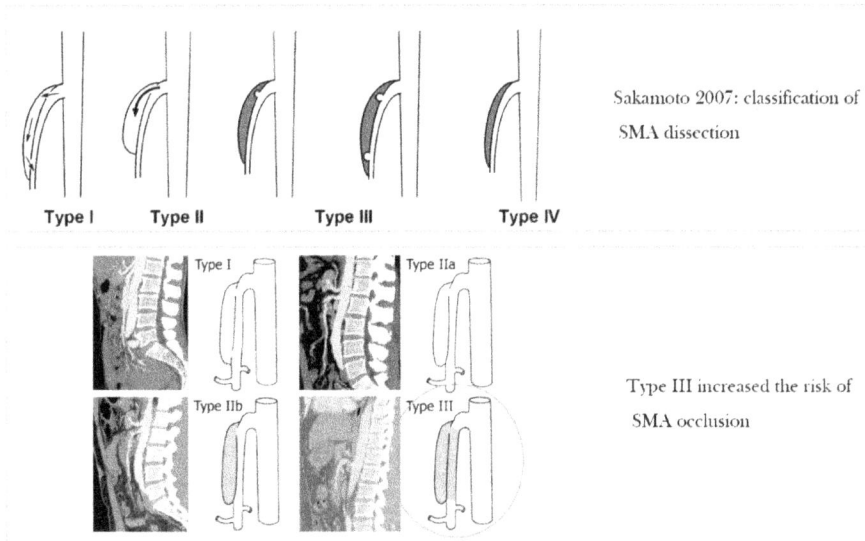

Figure 6.
The classification of SMA dissection. Slide courtesy to Dr. 李栋林浙江大学医学院附属第一医院血管外科.

Systematic review and meta-analysis for patients with spontaneous isolated superior mesenteric artery dissection also suggested conservative treatment [17–19].**Karaolanis2019**

2.13 Special scenario: combined celiac trunk and SMA disease

In our patient treated in December 2016, the patient had diffuse aorta atherosclerosis, with celiac trunk- hepatic artery and SMA ostial occlusion.

2.13.1 Chronic mesenteric ischemia involving both celiac trunk and SMA

For patients with chronic mesenteric ischemia due to occlusion of both celiac trunk and SMA, SMA revascularization alone may be adequate to improve symptoms [20].

2.14 Special scenario: ischemia: reperfusion syndrome

2.14.1 Reperfusion syndrome

Severe reperfusion syndrome after acute mesenteric ischemia revascularization has been reported. But optimal medical treatment has not been established **Robles–Martin2019.**

2.15 Recurrent superior mesenteric artery stent fracture

After successful stenting and salvage for acute mesenteric ischemia, stent fracture has been reported. This issue needs further study to establish the best treatment algorithm. Currently, we suggest following patients with abdominal contrast-enhanced CT to evaluate the patency of the stent **Robins 2019.**

3. Diagnosis of acute mesenteric ischemia

3.1 Initial phase- clinical challenges

The symptoms of acute mesenteric ischemia are described in most general text of most medical textbooks. We do not repeat the symptoms but wish to address the most common clinical challenges in the initial phase of diagnosis: after performing KUB plain film of CT angiography, it is still frequent to fail to proceed to invasive angiography due to multiple reasons: physicians do not familiar with invasive angiography, lack of staffs to perform emergent angiography, no bowel necrosis and surgeon wish to treat the patient conservatively. Following serum lactate level only detects the patients in irreversible bowel necrosis and is not beneficial providing chances of early salvage.

3.2 Computer tomography- CT

The axial, coronal, sagittal, and 3D reconstruction in advance is mandatory to be reviewed in the initial diagnostic phases. However, in patients with extensive aortic calcification and ostial calcification, care must be taken to interpret the lumen area and stenosis, because the lumen may be mis-interpretated as patent due to extensive ostial calficaition.

CT findings of bowel necrosis: no enhancement of bowel loop, pneumatosis intestinalis, aeroportia (**Figure 7**).

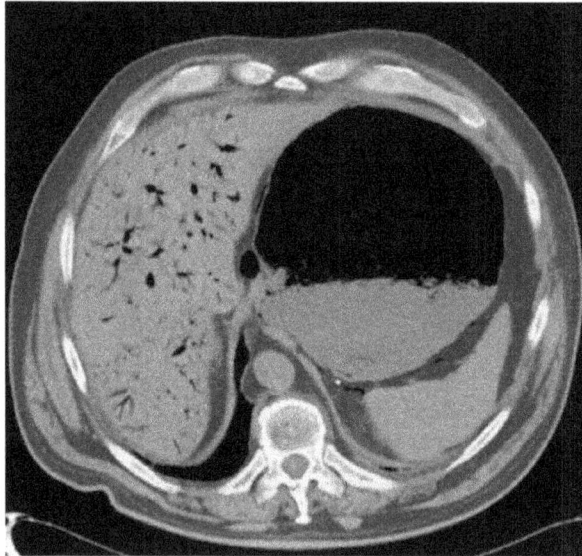

Figure 7.
The CT found extensive air within the portal venous system.

4. Consultation

4.1 Consultation process

After our index case, an interventional cardiologist (Mu-Yang Hsieh) wrote a draft. The draft was reviewed and completed by an interventional radiologist (Chih-Horng Wu). The interventional radiologist trained the interventional cardiologist to perform selective bowel angiography to reduce time delay in the emergency scenario.

The protocol was revised from the acute coronary syndrome protocol. For patients with evident bowel necrosis and peritoneal signs, direct consultation with a surgical team was mandatory (group 1 patients). The endovascular team was contacted after the surgical procedure. For patients with no evident bowel necrosis by CT, any team members can activate the protocol in the emergency department (group 2 patients). In suspected patients with possible CT findings (group 3 patients), the team votetd if proceeding with diagnostic angiography is beneficial to the patient **Figures 8–10**.

4.2 Surgical consultation

When the patient developed peritoneal signs or when bowel necrosis was evident by CT, the patient will be sent to the operation room first, and open

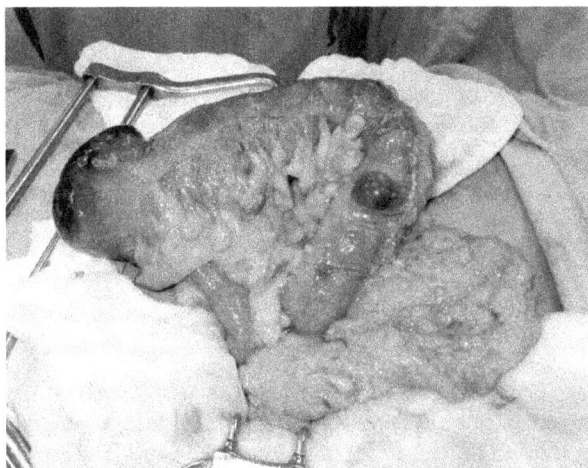

Figure 8.
During operation, direct manual examination after laparotomy confirms acute mesenteric ischemia with bowel necrosis.

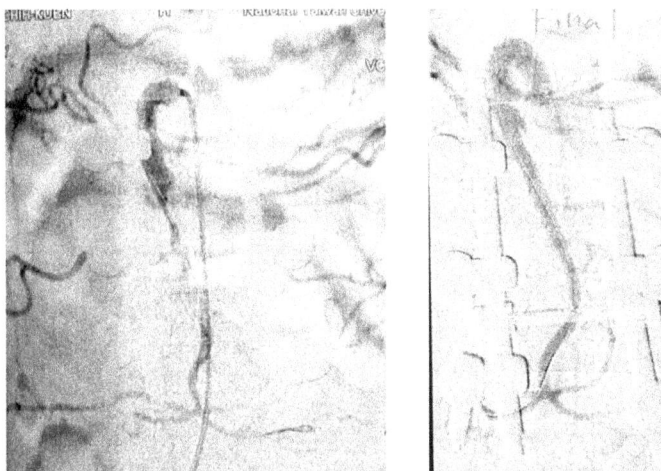

Figure 9.
During emergent angiography, total occlusion SMA was confirmed. The occlusion was re- canalized with a 0.014-INCH coronary wire, thrombosuction, and direct stenting. The abdominal pain completely resolved. No further surgical operation was needed.

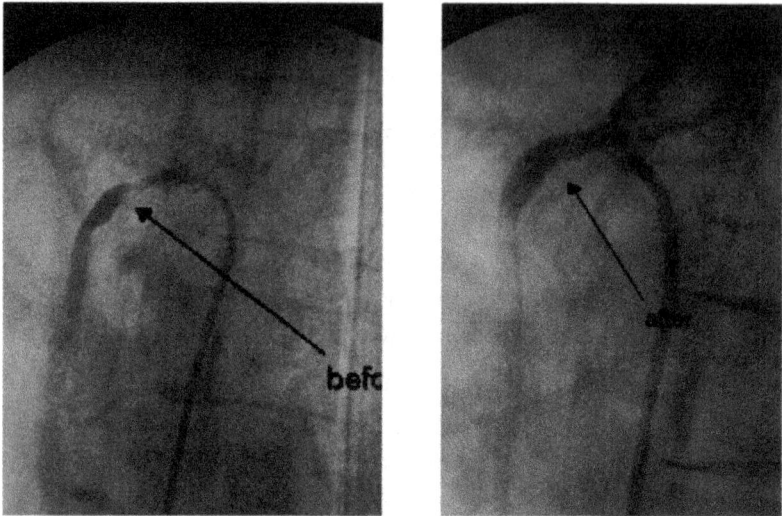

Figure 10.
Severe ostial stenosis of SMA. Treated with bare-metal stenting. The abdominal pain com- pletely resolved.

thrombectomy 及 retrograde open mesenteric stenting (ROMS) should be considered **Oderich 2018 Figure 11**.

4.2.1 Experience in the Hsinchu

Since 2016, we performed emergent angiography for case 9 and case 10 before the emergent open laparotomy. Direct stenting was performed on SMA. The potential benefit is to shorten the ischemic time (**Figures 12 and 13**).

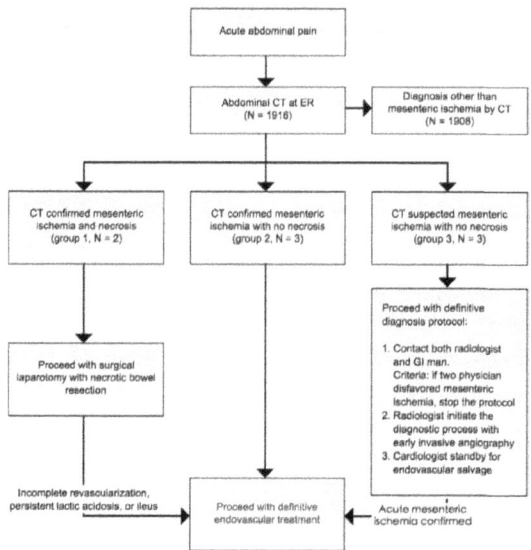

Figure 11.
The flow chart of consultation process according to CT imaging findings.

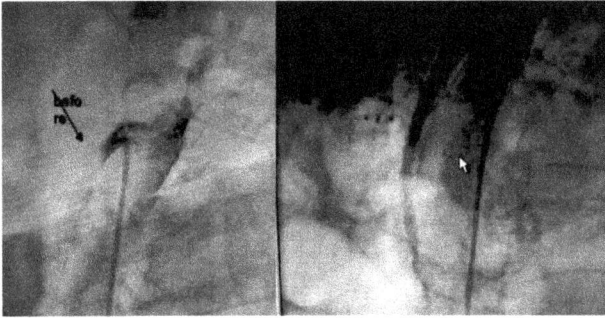

Figure 12.
Case 10: revascularization first! It is better with improved flow to jejunum and proximal ileum than SMA proximal total occlusion. During bowel resection, resect the ileocecal junction to ascending colon for ABOUT100 cm, with 200 cm viable small bowel saved after the revascularization.

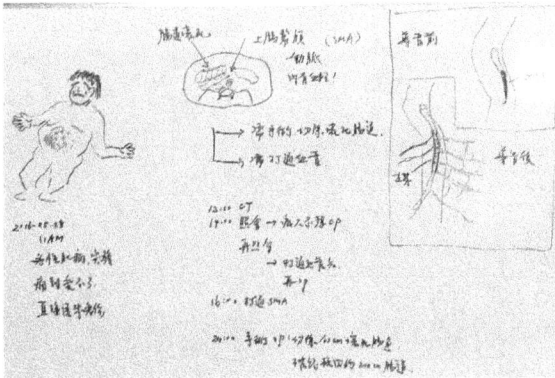

Figure 13.
Case illustration example. This illustration was made to make a thorough explanation to the patient and his family.

5. Critical statistics for patient explanation and the results pro- vided to the family for rapid briefing of acute mesenteric ischemia

Treatment results (historical results) were provided to the patient family at the emergency department.

- Angiographic (technical) success rate: 6/8 (75%)

- Survival at 30 days: 75%

- Survival at 7 days, In angiographic success patients: 100%

- Survival at 7 days, In angiographic failure patients: 0%

- Long-term follow-up survival at 2-YEAR: 50% (due to multiple comorbidities) (**Figure 14**).

Poster prepared and mounted in the emergency department and at the waiting area of intensive care units (**Figure 15**).

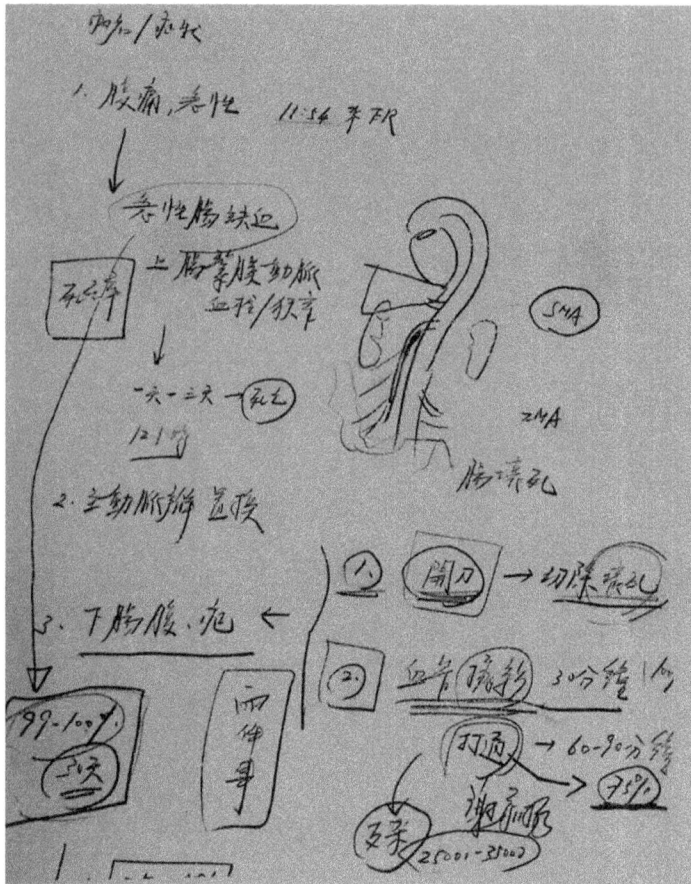

Figure 14.
The drawing of disease explanation. All the drawing was made in the emergency department.

6. Angiography and treatment

Abdominal angiography was performed emergently in the cath room (cardiology department) angiography room (radiology department). The vascular access was set with a 6-Fr sheath. To perform diagnostic angiography, a 5-Fr diagnostic catheter (RC-1 or JR) was used. In our protocol, the flow was rated using the coronary grading system: TIMI (thrombolysis in myocardial infarction) flow scale. Mesenteric artery disease was defined if there was diameter stenosis over 50%, and mesenteric artery occlusion was defined if there was 100% stenosis with 0 TIMI flow.

6.1 Endovascular treatment

Thrombosuction, balloon angioplasty, and stenting were performed sequentially or by the discretion of the interventional cardiologist. First, the femoral sheath was changed to a 7-Fr sheath (10 cm), and a guiding catheter (7-Fr JR4 or IMA) was used according to the angle between of SMA ostium and aorta after reviewing the sagittal view on the CT. For ostial lesion, a guide catheter with side hole was used. We usually give a bolus of heparin (3000–5000 U) to achieve activated clotting time of at least 250 seconds. A workhorse 0.014-INCH soft coronary wire was used to cross the lesion. With a dedicated coronary thrombosuction catheter, distal

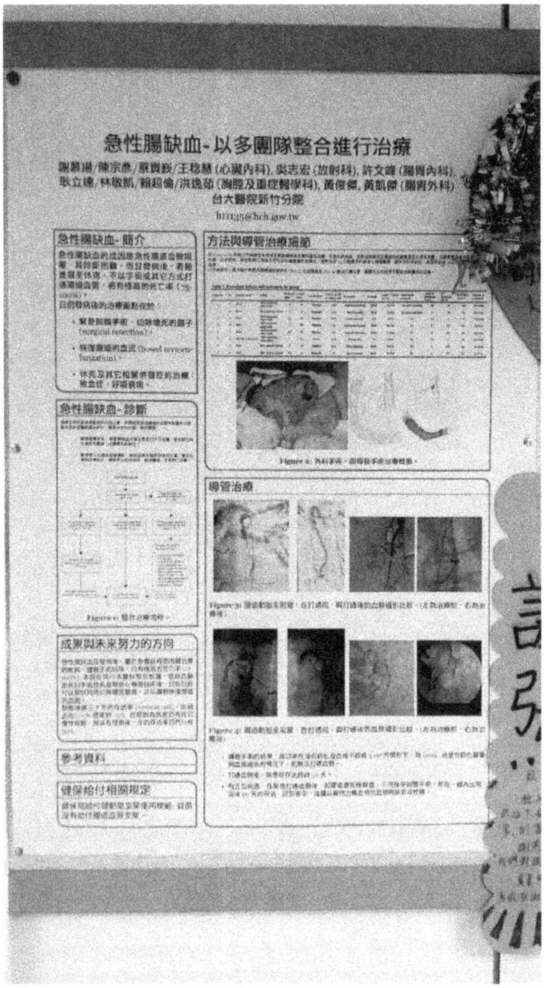

Figure 15.
The poster explaining the endovascular protocol for acute mesenteric ischemia. The poster was written in Chinese.

contrast injection can be done to confirm that true lumen was reached in cases with SMA occlusion. Thrombosuction was performed (Thrombuster, Terumo, Tokyo, Japan). Balloon angioplasty was done after successful establishment of antegrade flow. Ifpersistentt recoil or restenosis had been noted, the operator could perform bail-out stenting (usually with a coronary bare-metal stent. Thrombolytic agent was not used in our protocol because it was declined by our team (GI man). Because the National Health Insurance did not cover distal protection device in the treatment of acute mesenteric ischemia, the distal protection device was not used.

6.2 Procedure details

6.2.1 Percutaneous endovascular intervention

A coronary system with 0.014-INCH wire, balloon, and stents are used in our protocol. Usually, the vascular access is at the common femoral artery

(7 Fr sheath). We used a JR4 diagnostic coronary catheter with 0.035-inch wire (Terumo GlideWire) to perform diagnostic angiography. During the intervention, a 0.014-INCH coronary wire with length of 180 cm is used (Sion, BMW-U2).

6.2.2 Guiding catheter choices

The angle between SMA ostium and aorta can help to choose the suitable guide sheath or guiding catheter to engage SMA. The choices included angled sheath (6 or 7 Fr), IMA, or JR4 guide catheters.

6.2.3 Thrombosuction

Thrombosuction: we used coronary system, Thrombuster (6 Fr), or Export catheter.

6.2.4 Balloon angioplasty

Most commonly used balloons: Trek, Maverick, and Sapphire, with 6–8 atm.

6.2.5 Bail-out stenting

Bail-out stenting should be considered: when thrombosuction, or balloon angioplasty failed, stenting may still be tried.

Before performing bail-out stenting, we should always use thrombosuction catheter to perform distal injection in order to confirm the adequate distal landing zone.

Rotational Thrombectomy Device can be considered and has reported successful to salvage patients with acute mesenteric ischemia in a single center study [21].

7. Surgery

7.1 Inportant notices for surgeons

1. Surgery and revascularization are both mandatory to provide optimal survival chances in patients with extensive bowel necrosis.

2. For patients who received stenting to SMA before surgery, care must be taken not to manipulate the SMA forcefully to avoid inadvertent crush of the stent.

8. Post-stenting care

ICU care after the endovascular procedure is mandatory. The electrolyte, urine output, and arterial pressure are to be monitored. An infection specialist is consulted at the discretion of the critical care specialist. The general surgeon will check the abdominal physical exams to detect changes in peritoneal signs. As- pirin (100 mg) and clopidogrel (75 mg) are initiated if no bleeding is noted after overnight observation. For patients with atrial fibrillation, an oral anticoagulant is started at the discretion of the operator and the caring cardiologist.

8.1 Definition of treatment success

Important definition: [22].

• Primary clinical success was defined as complete resolution of symptoms.

• Partial clinical success was defined as resolution of some or most of the symptoms, but persistence of some symptoms after the procedure.

• Primary clinical failure was defined as the lack of any or minimal symptom relief.

• Technical success: the successful revascularization of all arteries that were treated in which there was less than a 30% residual diameter stenosis.

• Partial technical success per patient (who had multiple mesenteric arteries treated) was defined as at least one mesenteric artery treated successfully.

• Technical failure was defined as the inability to treat at least one mesenteric artery per patient

8.2 Antibiotics

Oral digestive decontamination: PO gentamicin 80 mg/day, PO metronidazole 1.5 g/day [23].
What Is the Role of Empiric Treatment for Suspected Invasive Candidiasis in Nonneutropenic Patients in the Intensive Care Unit?

8.2.1 Invasive candidiasis

Preferred empiric therapy for suspected candidiasis in non-neutropenic patients in the intensive care unit (ICU) is an echinocandin (caspofungin: loading dose of 70 mg, then 50 mg daily; micafungin: 100 mg daily; anidulafungin: loading dose of 200 mg, then 100 mg daily) (strong recommendation; moderate-quality evidence) [24].

8.3 ICU care

• Mandatory medical protocol: blood volume resuscitation, with mean arterial pressure > 65 mmHg, urine output > 0.5 ml/kg/hour.

• Curative unfractionated heparin therapy with aPTT 50–70 seconds.

• IV proton pump inhibitors: IV pantoprazole 80 mg/day

• Oxygen therapy

• Food resting, PN if prolonged > 5 days.

• Antibiotics: empirical, not prophylaxis. Tazocin and possible Candida coverage (no evidence of presence)

Important findings: In some patients with SMA and celiac trunk 100% occlusion, the patients can present with acute mesenteric ischemia. **Tables 4 and 5.**

No	Age	Sex	Comirbidities	CHADS2-VASc	Shock	Resting dyspnea	Food avoidance	Diarrhea	Nausea/ vomiting	Ileus, diffuse	Ileus, localized	Lactate (mmol/L)
1	79	Female	Cirrhosis, gout	2	+	+	–	–	–	–	+	8.8
2	61	Male	PAOD, ESRD, DM, dyslipidemia, smoking	2	+	–	–	+	+	–	+	2.5
3	74	Female	HTN, dyslipidemia, gout	2	–	–	–	+	–	–	+	1.7
4	72	Female	DM, HTN	3	–+	–	–	–	+	–	7.4	
5	63	Female	Afib, VHD, mechanical valve, CVA, DM, HTN, dyslipidemia	5	–	+	–	–	–	–	+	2.4
6	74	Female	CAD, old MI, PAOD, ESRD, DM, HTN, dyslipidemia	4	+	+	–	–	–	–	+	5
7	86	Male	CAD, Afib, VHD, DM, HTN	3	–	–	–	–	–	–	+	2.6
8	80	Female	CAD, ESRD, DM, HTN	4	–	–	+	–	–	–	+	1

Table 4.
Demographics, clinical characteristics, and presentation of acute abdominal pain of the study participants.

Category	No	Culprint vessel	Lesion	Diameter (mm)	Length (mm)	Calcification	Time from ER to angiography	Treatment	Stenting	Angio / Clinical success	Laparotomy required	Angio to Discharge (days)	F/U durations (days)	Survival at 30 days	Outcome at 12 montsh
1	1	SMA	100% occlusion, main trunk	4	28	Minimal	24.5	Aspiration/ stenting	BMS	Yes/Yes	Yes (after stenting)	45	33	Yes	Moratlity
1	6	SMA	50% stenosis, ostium	4	5	Moderate	12.1	Direct stenging	BMS	Yes/Yes	Yes (before stenting)	21	166	Yes	Moratlity
2	4	SMA	100% occlusion, main trunk	2.5	40	Minimal	16.3	Aspiration only	NA	No/No	No	NA	1	No	Mortality
2	5	SMA	100% occlusion, main trunk	4	30	Minimal	3.4	Aspiration/ stenting	BMS	Yes/Yes	No	2	341	Yes	Survival
2	7	SMA	100% occlusion, main trunk	4.5	50	Minimal	5.5	Aspiration/ stenting	BMS	Yes/Yes	No	3	187	Yes	Survival
3	2	SMA & celiac trunk	100% occlusion, from ostium	3	NA	Severe	11.9	Wiring only	NA	No/No	No	NA	1	No	Mortality

Category	No	Culprint vessel	Lesion	Diameter (mm)	Length (mm)	Calcification	Time from ER to angiography	Treatment	Stenting	Angio / Clinical success	Laparotomy required	Angio to Discharge (days)	F/U durations (days)	Survival at 30 days	Outcome at 12 montsh
3	3	IMA	80% stenosis, ostium	3	15	Minimal	22.2	Direct stenting	BMS	Yes/Yes	No	2	465	Yes	Survival
3	8	SMA	90% stenosis, ostium	4.5	8	Moderate	9	Direct stenting	BMS	Yes/Yes	No	2	90	Yes	Survival

Table 5.
Procedure details and outcomes, by group.

Author details

Mu-Yang Hsieh
National Taiwan University Hospital Hsinchu Branch Cardiovascular
Center/Critical Care Center, Taiwan

*Address all correspondence to: drake1128@gmail.com

IntechOpen

References

[1] Acosta S, Bjorck M. Acute thrombo-embolic occlusion of the superior mesenteric artery: A prospective study in a well defined population. European Journal of Vascular and Endovascular Surgery. 2003;**26**:179-183

[2] Blauw JT, Bulut T, Oderich GS, et al. Mesenteric vascular treatment 2016: From open surgical repair to endovascular revascularization. Best Practice & Research. Clinical Gastroenterology. 2017;**31**:75-84

[3] Karkkainen JM, Acosta S. Acute mesenteric ischemia (Part II) - Vascular and endovascular surgical approaches. Best Practice & Research. Clinical Gastroenterology. 2017;**31**:27-38

[4] Aboyans V, Ricco JB, Bartelink MEL, et al. 2017 ESC guidelines on the diagnosis and treatment of peripheral arterial diseases, in collaboration with the European Society for Vascular Surgery (ESVS): Document covering atherosclerotic disease of extracranial carotid and vertebral, mesen- teric, renal, upper and lower extremity arteries endorsed by: The European stroke organization (ESO)the task force for the diagnosis and treatment of peripheral arterial diseases of the Eu- ropean Society of Cardiology (ESC) and of the European Society for Vascular Surgery (ESVS). European Heart Journal. 1 Mar 2018;**39**(9):763-816. DOI: 10.1093/eurheartj/ehx095

[5] Campion EW, Clair DG, Beach JM. Mesenteric Ischemia. New England Journal of Medicine. 2016;**374**:959-968

[6] Kassahun WT, Schulz T, Richter O, et al. Unchanged high mortality rates from acute occlusive intestinal ischemia: Six year review. Langenbeck's Archives of Surgery. Mar 2008;**393**(2):163-171. DOI: 10.1007/s00423-007-0263-5. Epub 2008 Jan 3

[7] Schoots IG, Koffeman GI, Legemate DA, et al. Systematic review of survival after acute mesenteric ischaemia according to disease aetiology. The British Journal of Surgery. 2004;**91**:17-27

[8] Park WM, Cherry K, Chua HK, et al. Current results of open revascularization for chronic mesenteric ischemia: A standard for comparison. Journal of Vascular Surgery. 2002;**35**:853-859

[9] Erben Y, Protack CD, Jean RA, et al. Endovascular interventions decrease length of hospitalization and are cost-effective in acute mesenteric ischemia. Journal of Vascular Surgery. Aug 2018;**68**(2):459-469. DOI: 10.1016/j.jvs.2017.11.078

[10] Zhang Z, Wang D, Li G, et al. Endovascular treatment for acute thromboembolic occlusion of the superior mesenteric artery and the outcome comparison between endovascular and open surgical treatments: A retrospective study. BioMed Research International. 2017;**2017**:1-10

[11] Lim S, Halandras PM, Bechara C, et al. Contemporary Management of Acute Mesenteric Ischemia in the endovascular era. Vascular and Endovascular Surgery. 2019;**53**:42-50

[12] Forbrig R, Renner P, Kasprzak P, et al. Outcome of primary percutaneous stent-revascularization in patients with atherosclerotic acute mesenteric ischemia. Acta Radiologica. 2017;**58**:311-315

[13] Miura Y, Araki T, Terashima M, et al. Mechanical recanalization for acute embolic occlusion at the origin of the superior mesenteric artery. Vascular and Endovascular Surgery. 2017;**51**:91-94

[14] Mendes BC, Oderich GS, Tallarita T, et al. Superior mesenteric artery stenting using embolic pro- tection device for treatment of acute or chronic mesenteric ischemia. Journal of Vascular Surgery. Oct 2018;**68**(4):1071-1078. DOI: 10.1016/j.jvs.2017.12.076. Epub 2018 Apr 21

[15] Morbi AH, Nordon IM. Emergency revascularisation in a patient with acute mesenteric is- chaemia: The role of open revascularisation and compensatory blood flow. Acta Chirurgica Belgica. 2016;**116**:234-238

[16] Gobble RM, Brill ER, Rockman CB, et al. Endovascular treatment of spontaneous dissections of the superior mesenteric artery. Journal of Vascular Surgery. 2009;**50**:1326-1332

[17] Loeffler JW, Obara H, Fujimura N, et al. Medical therapy and intervention do not improve un- complicated isolated mesenteric artery dissection outcomes over observation alone. Journal of Vascular Surgery. 2017;**66**:202-208

[18] Kimura Y, Kato T, Inoko M. Outcomes of treatment strategies for isolated spontaneous dis- section of the superior mesenteric artery: A systematic review. Annals of Vascular Surgery. 2018;**47**:284-290

[19] Liu Q, Li TJ, Zeng R, et al. Effect of adequate Anticoagulantion therapy on the outcome of Spon- taneous isolated dissection of superior mesenteric artery. Zhongguo Yi Xue Ke Xue Yuan Xue Bao. 2018;**40**:21-25

[20] Goldman MP, Reeve TE, Craven TE, et al. Endovascular treatment of chronic mesenteric ischemia in the setting of occlusive superior mesenteric artery lesions. Annals of Vascular Surgery. 2017;**38**:29-35

[21] Freitas B, Bausback Y, Schuster J, et al. Thrombectomy devices in the treatment of acute Mesen- teric

ischemia: Initial single-center experience. Annals of Vascular Surgery. 2018;**51**:124-131

[22] Turba UC, Saad WE, Arslan B, et al. Chronic mesenteric ischaemia: 28-YEAR experience of endovas- cular treatment. European Radiology. 2012;**22**:1372-1384

[23] Roussel A, Castier Y, Nuzzo A, et al. Revascularization of acute mesenteric ischemia after creation of a dedicated multidisciplinary center. Journal of Vascular Surgery. 2015;**62**:1251-1256

[24] Pappas PG, Kauffman CA, Andes DR, et al. Executive summary: Clinical practice guideline for the Management of Candidiasis: 2016 update by the Infectious Diseases Society of America. Clinical Infectious Diseases. 2016;**62**:409-417

Chapter 4

Choosing the Right Guidewire: The Key for a Successful Revascularization

Daniel Brandão

Abstract

Even though frequently less considered, the guidewires are the most fundamental tools to track throughout the vessels, to cross stenoses or occlusions, and to be able to deliver the desired therapy to the selected vessel. In this chapter entitled "Choosing the Right Guidewire: The Key for a Successful Revascularization," the following issues will be thoroughly described: how the guidewires are built and why it is so important to be aware of it; why are there so many different guidewires; what are the possible applications for each guidewire; how to choose the right guidewire in every situation; techniques to cross a stenosis and a chronic total occlusion.

Keywords: guidewire, core, tip, stenosis, occlusion

1. Introduction

Even though frequently less considered, the guidewires are the most fundamental tools to track throughout the vessels, to cross stenoses or occlusions, and to be able to deliver the desired therapy to the target lesion of a given vessel. A thorough knowledge of how they are built and in what way this impacts on their specific characteristics and applications is crucial for any vascular specialist who wishes to succeed. In fact, considering the vast number of options, a correct choice and utilization of a guidewire can frequently be the difference between success and failure of a revascularization, avoiding many possible complications that can jeopardize the final result.

2. General characteristics

2.1 Length

The selection of a guidewire with a correct length can be very relevant to adequately reach and treat the target vessel. For this decision, distance from the access to the vessel to be treated and the shaft length of the sheaths and catheters to be used (either if it is a diagnostic catheter, a balloon catheter, or a delivery device of a stent or a stent graft) needs to be considered. In fact, this apparently less relevant subject may threaten the entire procedure.

Depending on the manufacturer, guidewires can range from 80 to 450 cm. Additionally, some guidewires may allow the connection of an extension during the procedure. This is particularly the case when a coronary guidewire is used as it is designed for rapid exchange devices.

There is a trick that can help in extreme circumstances and as bailout option only. During the removal of a catheter from inside the patient, it is possible to connect an inflation syringe device to the guidewire port of the catheter, just after losing the guidewire, and inflate inside the port, which will keep the guidewire in place. It is crucial to perform this maneuver under fluoroscopy as the guidewire may move forward and the external tip can even migrate and be lost inside the patient.

2.2 Diameter

Even if there are several diameters available, the most commonly used guidewires to cross stenoses and occlusions in peripheral arteries have 0.014″, 0.018″, or 0.035″ in diameter. At this point, it will be relevant to recall the relation between the different units used in endovascular devices, as so: 1 French (F) = 1/3 millimeter = 0.013 inches. It is quite obvious that the thicker the guidewire, the stiffer it is and the more support it allows, even if the core material of it is also very relevant for those properties.

They are several factors that someone should keep in mind when choosing the diameter of a guidewire:

- The vessel(s) to be tracked. The smaller the vessels to be tracked, the smaller the guidewire should be. For instance, in the iliac arteries or in the aorta, the guidewires usually used are 0.035″ in diameter, as it is when a crossover at the aortic bifurcation is necessary. In tibial vessels, 0.018″ or 0.014″ guidewires are usually the preferred diameters and in the delicate foot arteries, the 0.014″ guidewires are the rule. Another issue is the distance from the access to the target vessel(s). Logically, the longer the distance, the more support will be needed and the thicker the guidewire will need to be.

- The target vessel(s). As for the vessels to be tracked, the smaller the vessel, the thinner the guidewire should usually be.

- The kind of lesion(s) to be treated (stenosis versus occlusion). Even if occlusions are usually more difficult to cross, some stenoses can be particularly challenging. In fact very tight heavily calcified stenoses may initially allow the passage of a thicker guidewire, but can preclude the crossing of catheters with the corresponding caliber. In these situations, a downsizing of the guidewire diameter is required. For instance, in tibial vessels of diabetic patients, particularly those with end-stage renal disease, calcified stenoses can be crossed with a 0.018″ guidewire, but frequently, the balloon catheter is not able to cross impelling the change to a 0.014″ system (**Figure 1**).

- The devices planned to be used and their respective platform.

- The support needed to deliver the intended devices.

- The operator's preference. In many instances, several guidewires with different diameters can be used. This will depend on the experience of the operator with a particular guidewire or the institutional availability. Most of the times, there is no right or wrong as long as the aim of the intervention is successfully fulfilled.

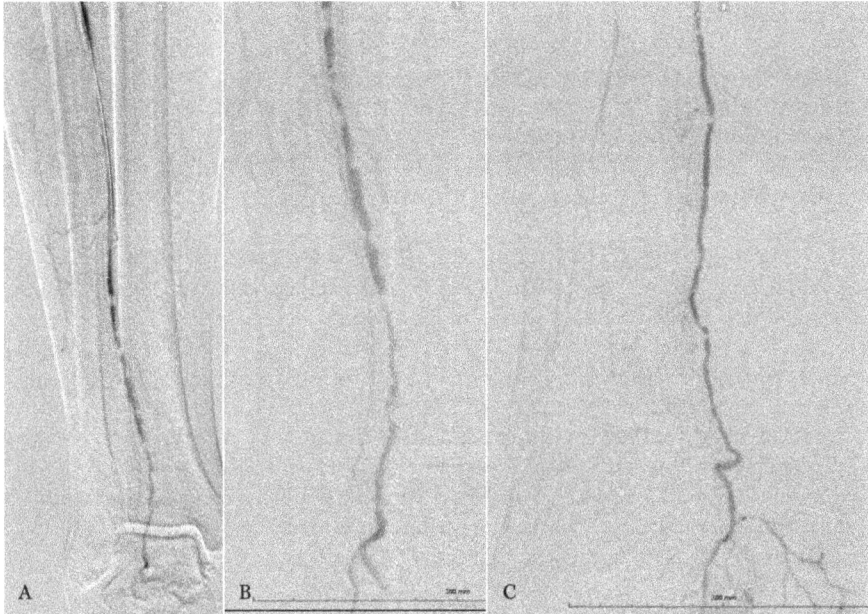

Figure 1.
A, B—Anterior tibial artery with very calcified and tight stenoses. C—Posterior tibial artery of the same patient (diabetic and on hemodialysis). The stenoses were successfully crossed and treated with angioplasty with a 0.014" guidewire.

2.3 Stiffness

There is no clearly accepted nomenclature that can reproductively relate a word or a group of words to the stiffness of a guidewire. As so, it is possible to find several guidewires with the label stiff, extra stiff, super stiff, or even ultra-stiff, without any objective information of its real stiffness. Flexural modulus is an engineering parameter related to a wire's resistance to bending (**Figure 2**). This measure is rarely displayed on the guidewire packaging or within the catalog [1]. Yet, it represents an objective method to quantify the stiffness of a guidewire.

This property is more frequently used to describe the body of the guidewire, but its use in the description of the tip of the guidewire can be very useful too. The stiffer the body of a guidewire is, the more support it will allow to deliver the intended endovascular devices to the target vessel. On the other end, a higher stiffness of the body reduces the ability of the guidewire to track the vessel tree. Concerning the tip, a higher stiffness increases the penetration capacity, but also turns the tip more aggressive to vessel wall increasing the risk of dissection or perforation.

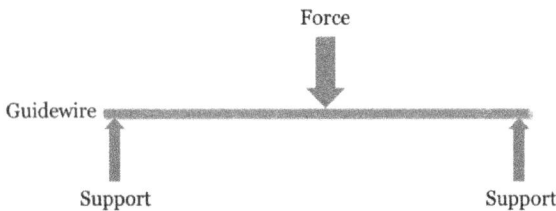

Figure 2.
Generically, the guidewire is supported at two points that are equidistant to a third point where a vertical force is applied. The force needed to bend the guidewire to a given extent determines its stiffness.

2.4 Trackability

It represents the capacity of a guidewire to navigate through the arterial tree, especially through curves of tortuous vessels. As so, floppier guidewires have a better trackability than stiffer guidewires.

2.5 Crossability

It characterizes the ability of a guidewire to easily cross a lesion without buckling or kinking. Several features of the guidewire can optimize this capacity, depending on whether it is a stenosis or a chronic total occlusion.

2.6 Pushability

Pushability can be defined by the percentage or amount of a given forward force applied to the proximal end of the guidewire that is transmitted to the distal end of the guidewire. Usually, the stiffer and broader the guidewire, the more pushability it gives. This characteristic is particularly relevant in crossing long and/or calcified chronic total occlusions, either in an intraluminal or subintimal way.

2.7 Torqueability

Torqueability represents the ability to apply a given rotational force at the proximal end of the guidewire and have that force transmitted efficiently and with the less delay possible, to achieve proper control of the distal tip. This feature is very relevant to determine the path of the guidewire and, consequently, to navigate inside the arterial tree (for instance, to go from the popliteal artery to the anterior tibial artery without a curved catheter) or to cross lesions. Torqueability is very dependent on the material used in the core and the distance from the access to the tip of the guidewire. As an example, guidewires with a stainless-steel core lose most their torqueability when used in a crossover fashion.

3. Composition

A basic knowledge of the engineering aspects of the guidewire technology is quite relevant to understand more thoroughly how a given guidewire is expected to behave in different conditions.

A guidewire has essentially four major components (**Figures 3** and **4**):

1. the body;

2. the tip;

3. the cover of both the body and tip;

4. the final coating of both the body and tip.

3.1 Core

A guidewire has a core that goes all the way through the body and finishes at the tip, where it may or may not reach the end of the guidewire (**Figure 5**). The core can be made of nitinol (alloy of nickel and titanium), stainless steel, or another metallic alloy. Nitinol allows more flexibility, memory (ability to maintain the original shape), and resistance to bending. Stainless steel increases the stiffness of the

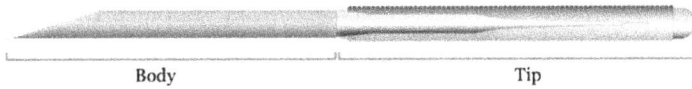

Figure 3.
Basic composition of a guidewire.

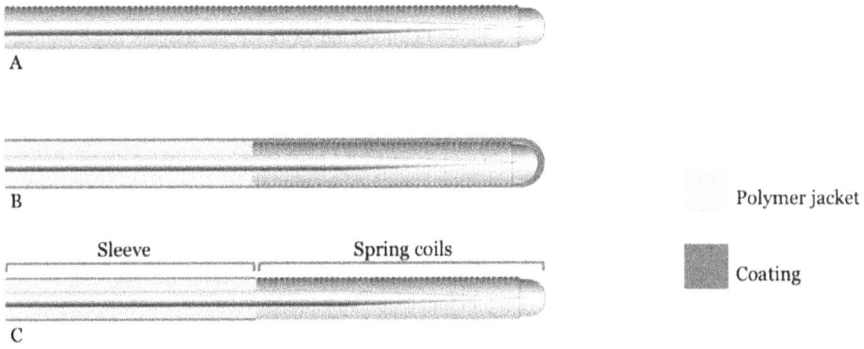

Figure 4.
A—Spring coils design. B—Guidewire with a complete polymer jacket and coating. C—Hybrid covering.

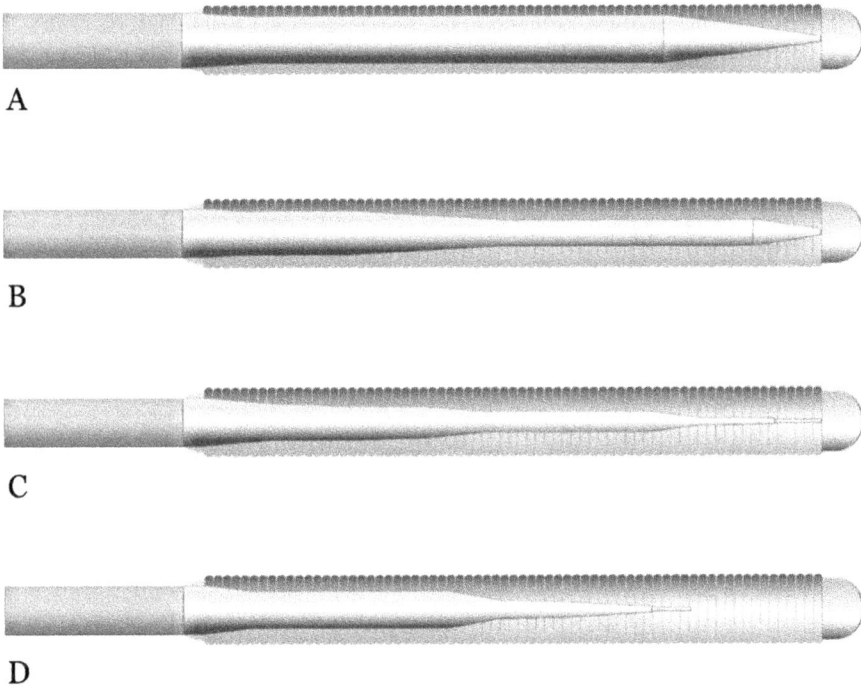

Figure 5.
A, B, C—Core-to-tip design. The core taper is longer and segmented in B and C. D – Shaping ribbon design.

guidewire, but is less resistant to bending, so it is easier to irreversibly kink a guide-wire with a stainless-steel core than a guidewire with a nitinol core. Other alloys will provide intermediate characteristics. Some guidewires may also have hybrid cores with stainless steel in the body and nitinol in the tip. In addition to its composition, its thickness straightforwardly corresponds to its stiffness: the thicker the core, the greater the stiffness and support. Therefore, the core is decisive for the behavior of the guidewire concerning its stiffness, torqueability, pushability, and trackability.

3.2 Tip

There are essentially two main inner designs concerning the tip (**Figure 5**): the core finishes at the end of the tip in a variable tapered format (core-to-tip design) [2]. In this configuration, the tip has more pushability and torque, a higher penetration capacity, and a better tactile feel (see below). On the other hand, the tip is more prone to inadvertently perforate a vessel, to prolapse to an undesired vessel during tracking the arterial tree (**Figure 6A**) and to be irreversibly damaged (especially if the core is made of stainless steel). The length of the core taper and its configuration in a continuous or segmented design will enhance or attenuate the enumerated characteristics (**Figure 5A–C**).

The core does not reach the end of the tip (shaping ribbon design) [2]. With this configuration, the end of the tip is wrapped in a small flexible metal ribbon, providing the continuity of the guidewire (**Figure 5D**). This design provides a less aggressive and flexible tip, less prone to prolapse (**Figure 6B**), easier to shape, though at the cost of a less tip torque control.

The outer diameter of conventional guidewires is usually the same throughout its length. However, in more dedicated devices, the tip has a progressive reduction of the diameter (tapered tip design—**Figure 7**), going, for instance, from 0.014″ to 0.009″ [2]. This characteristic increases the penetration capacity but turns the tip much more aggressive and prone to vessel perforation. These guidewires are almost exclusively utilized in chronic total occlusions and should be handled with extreme care.

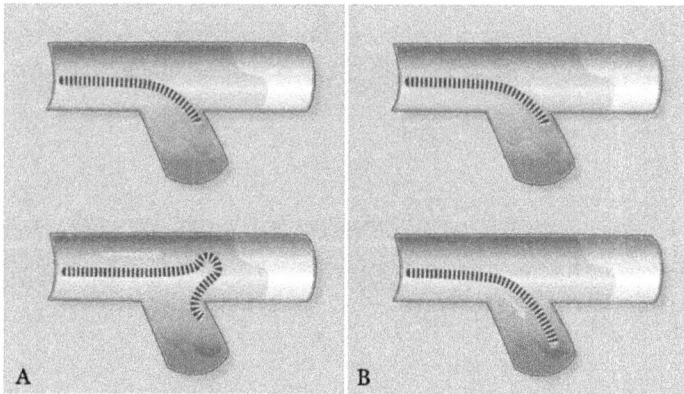

Figure 6.
A—A guidewire with a core-to-tip design has more difficulties in tracking the arterial tree and can prolapse to an undesired vessel. B—A guidewire with a shaping ribbon design tracks the intended vessel much more easily. Arrows indicate the natural direction of each guidewire.

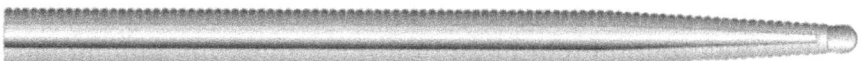

Figure 7.
An example of a tapered tip design.

3.3 Cover

The core of the guidewire is usually covered either by coils or by a polymer component (**Figure 4**). When all the core is surrounded only by spring coils (spring coils design), it enhances tactile feel (see below), but adds friction when navigating the arterial tree, reducing trackability. However, this additional friction tends to stabilize the wire distally to the target lesion, making the guidewire less prone to move backward or forward. On the other hand, a polymer jacket along all the guidewire including the tip provides a very smooth surface improving trackability at the cost of losing tactile feel. Some guidewires have a hybrid covering or polymer covering all the body but leaving the coils of the tip naked, also referred to as "sleeves" [3]. This configuration allows good trackability of the body maintaining tactile feel mostly intact.

3.4 Coating

Most of contemporary guidewires have a thin hydrophilic or hydrophobic coating applied at the final manufacturing process (**Figure 4**). Hydrophilic coating (e.g., polyethylene oxide or polyvinyl pyrolidone) needs water to be activated and to become slippery, but once wet, it allows an extremely low coefficient of friction [4]. As a result, it makes vessels easier to track and stenoses simpler to cross but leads to a decreased tactile feel, increasing the risk of dissection or perforation. Paradoxically, if a guidewire with hydrophilic coating gets dry, it loses lubricity and can get stuck, for instance, inside a catheter. Conversely, hydrophobic coatings (e.g., polytetrafluoroethylene or silicones) do not require water for activation [4]. As their name indicates, they repel water and create a smooth, "wax-like" surface [3]. Hydrophobic coating reduces friction but leads to a less slippery guidewire with enhanced tactile feel. Frequently, hydrophobic coatings are applied to guidewire bodies to facilitate movement inside plastic catheters [4]. Nevertheless, both coatings can coexist in a single guidewire, allowing their respective specific characteristics to be present either at the tip or throughout the body. In some configurations, even the tip can have both coatings, for instance, hydrophobic at the end for tactile feel and tip control purposes and hydrophilic intermediate segment for smooth crossing. Moreover, both hydrophilic and hydrophobic coatings may chafe or degrade with use [4]. This can account for the deterioration in wire performance at times noted during long procedures, particularly when wires are working through areas of severe tortuosity and friction or after numerous device exchanges [4]. This can even lead the guidewire to get fixed inside the catheter, forcing both devices to be removed as one piece, jeopardizing the therapy of the targeted vessel.

4. Specific characteristics

Even though, they are common to all guidewires used in endovascular procedures, the characteristics that will be discussed here are much more relevant in the 0.014″ and 0.018″ guidewires.

4.1 Tactile feel

It reports to the ability of a guidewire in transmitting tactile information from its tip to the hands of the interventionist. Even though it is a relatively subjective property, the possibility of the interventionist to feel the behavior of the tip when tracking vessels or crossing lesions (e.g., the tip goes freely or finds resistance) can help avoiding complications and improving results.

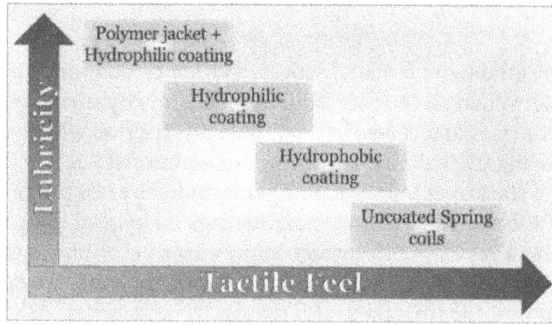

Figure 8.
Components combination influencing the relationship between lubricity and tactile feel.

There is an inverse relationship between lubricity and tactile feel (**Figure 8**). Moreover, specific features can enhance tactile feel such as the core-to-tip design and the spring coil design.

4.2 Tip load

The tip load represents the stiffness of the tip and is defined by the force needed to deflect to bend the tip 2 mm when the wire is fixed 10 mm above its end (**Figure 9**). It is a quite well-defined and reproducible parameter and therefore a comparable property. But as it is expressed in grams, it can generate confusion making some to think that the guidewire has effectively added weights at the tip. The tip load of the 0.014″ and 0.018″ guidewires utilized in peripheral interventions can range from 0.5 up to 35 g or more. The higher the tip load, the more aggressive the tip is. The lower it is, the softer and atraumatic it is.

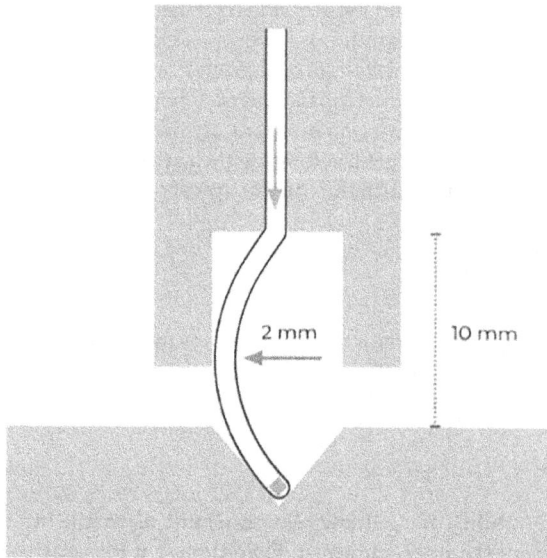

Figure 9.
Tip load test.

4.3 Penetration capacity

The penetration capacity can be defined by the perpendicular force exerted over a defined area (i.e., pressure). It will depend on the tip load and the profile of the tip. For the same tip load, a guidewire that has a tapered tip will have a much higher penetration capacity than a more conventional nontapered tip. Additionally, adding a catheter (either a balloon catheter or a support catheter) very close to the end of the tip also adds penetration capacity as it prevents the tip to bend.

4.4 Shape, shapeability, and shape retention

Most of the 0.035″ guidewires used in peripheral interventions come in a preshaped format from the manufacturer. The more common available shapes are straight, angled, and J-shaped. The latter is the least traumatic. As so, it can be the best guidewire to use to deliver the intended devices to a target vessel. It can also be quite useful in tracking throughout a previously placed patent stent because the tip will not get stuck in the struts of the stent, neither will go between the stent and the vessel wall. Straight tips are more adequate to cross occlusions and angled tips to track vessels and to cross stenoses.

On the other hand, the vast majority of the 0.014″ and 0.018″ guidewires available for peripheral purposes comes in a straight shape and needs to be shaped. As so, shapeability characterizes the capacity of the guidewire tip to be angulated and shaped by the interventionist and shape retention represents its ability to maintain the intended shape over time [3]. These properties depend on the tip design and materials. Accordingly, a core-to-tip design with a core made of stainless steel is particularly easy and accurate to be shaped, but almost impossible to be reshaped. Conversely, nitinol core makes the tip more difficult to be shaped because it tends to return to its original form (memory) but is more reshapeable.

The tip of the GW can be shaped using the puncture needle (for moderately angulated curves), with the non-cutting edge of the blade (for sharp angulations) or with the inserter (for both) (Videos 1 and 2, https://bit.ly/3jPF7aj).

The desired shape depends on the primary purpose the guidewire will be used (**Figure 10**). Moderately angled continuous curves are very useful to track throughout the artery tree or to select a target vessel (**Figure 10A**). Several sharp angulations may help in selecting arteries with an acute takeoff such as the anterior tibial artery

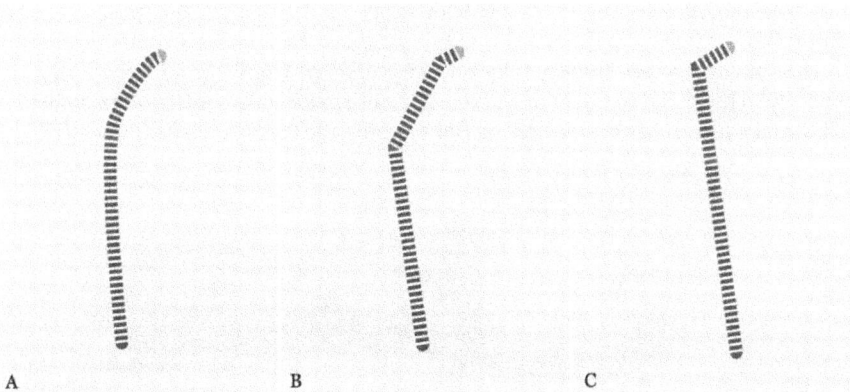

A   B   C

Figure 10.
Tip shaping. A—Moderately angled continuous curve. B—Two sharp angles. C—Very short sharply angled curve.

(**Figure 10B**). A very short sharply angled curve (usually no more than 1 mm) is intended to perform forceful and well-controllable drilling (**Figure 10C**).

5. Guidewire selection

An accurate knowledge of the discussed characteristics of each guidewire will permit the proper choice for every specific situation and also to create an adequate local laboratory portfolio. In practice, a vascular interventionist will rather need to thoroughly master a relatively small number of guidewires, instead of scarcely knowing many.

The purpose of guidewires in a peripheral procedure can be summarized as:

• getting to the target vessel;

• crossing the target lesion;

• give support to deliver the intended devices to the target lesion in a safely way.

Most of the interventionists have one or two "workhorse" guidewires, which are the guidewires that will be chosen to initiate the procedure and get to the target vessel. Their common characteristics are: good trackability and torqueability to navigate throughout the arterial tree, correct body stiffness to deliver catheters and sheaths to the intended vessel, and a tip as atraumatic as possible. They can also be used as an initial approach to the target lesion.

One additional aspect to take into account when choosing a guidewire is the catheter that will be also used. As such, for stenoses and some occlusions in larger vessels, such as the iliac arteries, an angled diagnostic or support catheter can be preferred to guide the tip of the guidewire to the center of the vessel, avoiding a subintimal track. Meanwhile, a straight support catheter or a balloon catheter would be the primary option for most of the stenoses and for occlusions in smaller vessels such as the tibial arteries.

5.1 Basic rules for guidewire manipulation

One of the best friends of a vascular interventionist is the torquer (**Figure 11**). It is the most proper manner to control the orientation of the guidewire tip. Therefore, its utilization is of utmost relevance in tracking difficult anatomies or in crossing challenging lesions (for instance, if the drilling technique is to be employed).

After having crossed the target lesion, the guidewire should be advanced very smoothly to the distal segment of the vessel. Confirmation through contrast injection that the true lumen has been reached after crossing the lesion is a basic but essential

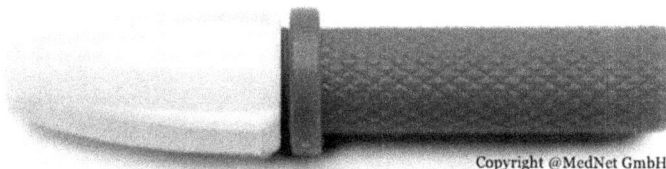

Copyright @MedNet GmbH

Figure 11.
Example of a torquer.

step. If a guidewire with a very aggressive tip was used to cross the lesion, it should be replaced by a much safer guidewire with good body stiffness for support (frequently the initial workhorse guidewire is adequate for this intent), sometimes after having shaped the tip as a loop (J-shaped like). During the delivery of the intended devices to the target lesion, it is of paramount importance to avoid inadvertent retraction of the guidewire, particularly after a complex crossing step and to prevent back and forth or shaking motion of the guidewire. That is why the tip of the guidewire should be on sight at almost all times. In summary, the two goals are: to secure the access to the target vessel and lesion; to avoid any trauma to the distal intact vessels.

5.2 Crossing the target lesion

The opening "workhorse" guidewire can be used in an initial attempt to cross the target lesion. Nevertheless, in many circumstances, a more dedicated guidewire will be required.

5.2.1 Crossing a stenosis

To cross a stenosis, it is perceptibly fundamental to stay intraluminal. For that purpose, the guidewire does not need to have increased stiffness, pushability, or penetration capacity. The tip should probably be hydrophilic as tactile feel is less relevant in those situations, and this can also improve the crossability of the guide-wire. The tip is typically shaped in soft curve (**Figure 10A**), to be directed to the opposite direction of the stenosis. Specifically in tibial vessels, a 0.014″ guidewire can be preferable as in the case showed in **Figure 1**.

5.2.2 Crossing a chronic total occlusion

A chronic total occlusion is generally defined as an occluded artery of 3 months duration or longer [5]. When the vascular interventionist faces a chronic total occlusion, the best guidewire is obviously the one that successfully crosses the lesion. Nevertheless, there are several issues to consider in an attempt to cross a chronic total occlusion:

- The target artery. In fact, some arteries can be quite challenging to recanalize. For instance, an occlusion of the anterior tibial artery from its origin is, most of the times, very challenging to cross anterogradely because of the difficulty to engage the ostium. In those circumstances, adjuvant retrograde approach can be very helpful.

- The length of the occlusion. Longer occlusions are more difficult to cross and involve additional struggle to keep the guidewire in an intraluminal track. Moreover, the guidewire should have a stiffer body to support the crossing of a balloon or a support catheter, and it can also frequently require segmental pre-dilatations.

- The associated calcification. Depending on its length, location (entry point of the occlusion and/or in its core), and whether it is concentric or eccentric, calcification can greatly complicate the crossing of an occlusion or the reentry after a subintimal path. It also increases the risk of complications such as perforations or ateroembolization. On another hand, medial calcification can occasionally help in defining the limits of the vessel and consequently can guide the interventionist to stay intraluminal.

- Visible run-off. As a rule, the end of the chronic total occlusion should be clearly defined. Nevertheless, in some instances, such as in tibial vessels with very poor collateralization, it may not be initially adequately outlined and only appears after having crossed the occlusion.

5.2.3 Sliding technique

This technique is particularly indicated for engaging softer chronic total occlusions with microchannels [6]. It is frequently the first approach. For that intent, the initial "workhorse" guidewire with a soft hydrophilic tip and a body with some stiffness can be the option as reduced surface friction enhances passage through the chronic total occlusion core. The tip should initially be shaped in a single, long shallow bend (**Figure 10A**), and movement consists of simultaneous smooth tip rotation and gentle probing. But during the crossing, the intervention-ist should stay vigilant, as the guidewire has reduced tactile feel and typically advances with minimal resistance, frequently resulting in inadvertent entry to the subintimal space [7].

5.2.4 Drilling technique

If the sliding technique fails after a few attempts (one should not insist on this technique as it is easy to create several subintimal tracks that will jeopardize a desirable intra-luminal crossing), then the drilling technique should be tried. In this technique, a guidewire with a core-to-tip design with an uncovered tip should be preferred to enhance tactile feel. The tip is bended in a very short extension (**Figure 10C**) and clockwise and counterclockwise rotations of the guidewire are performed while the tip is pushed modestly against the chronic total occlusion (**Figure 12**). The important issue in this technique is that one does not push the guidewire very hard. Placing the balloon or the support catheter very close to the tip increases the penetration capacity. If the tip of the guidewire does not advance any more with gentle pushing, it is by far better to exchange for a stiffer tip and body guidewire, rather than continue pushing. If one pushes the wire hard, it will easily go into the subintimal space. Yet, when a stiffer guidewire is used, it may be difficult to perceive whether the tip has been engaged in the true or in a false lumen inside the chronic total occlusion. The movement of the tip may help in distin-guishing one from the other. Typically, when the guidewire is in the subadventitial space, the tip budges markedly. Tactile feel from the guidewire during pullback can also aid as true lumen usually offers higher resistance. This technique has an increased risk of perforation, especially when using stiff tips guidewires [7].

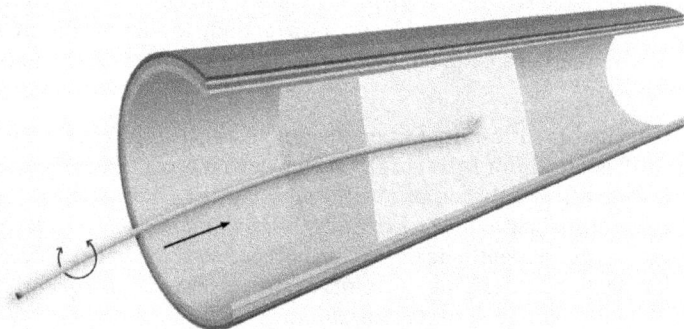

Figure 12.
Drilling technique. Adapted from [7].

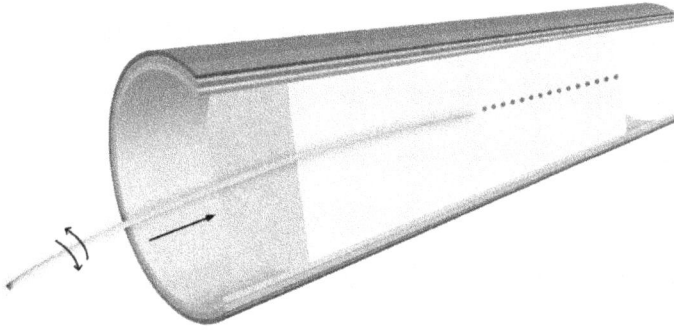

Figure 13.
Penetrating technique. Adapted from [7].

5.2.5 Penetrating technique

The penetration technique comes next if the drilling technique does not succeed or when the interventionist has a chronic total occlusion with very calcified cap. In this technique, the preferred guidewires have a very aggressive tip (core to-tip design, uncovered tapered tip, with increased tip load, and a subsequent high penetration capacity) and a relatively stiff body. The tip shape is essentially straight, and a less rotational tip motion and a more direct forward probing is used in comparison to the drilling technique (**Figure 13**). Again, placing the balloon or the support catheter very close to the tip increases the penetration capacity and reduces the propensity of the tip to bend. Additionally, the distal target must be clearly identified and careful monitoring of the progressive guidewire advancement should be done. The guidewires employed in this technique should not be used to deliver the intended devices to the target lesion as the tip can easily damage the distally intact vessels. It is a technique with a particularly augmented risk of complications [7].

5.2.6 Subintimal technique

It is usually the last technique to be employed, even if it can be a first option in specific situations such as very long chronic total occlusions. For this technique, a guidewire with a stiff body and a soft short tip with hydrophilic coating is usually preferable. The short tip allows a short loop. After having created the loop, the guidewire is advanced to the end of the occlusion. To reenter into the true lumen, the loop has to be undone. Sometimes, the guidewire needed to be exchanged to a guidewire with a reduced diameter (if the initial guidewire was not a 0.014″ guidewire), with an uncovered tip (to increase the tactile feel and reduce the tendency to stay in the subintimal space that a hydrophilic tips has), a good torqueability, and an angled shaped tip (to be able to direct this one to the true lumen). Sometimes moving the balloon or the support catheter and the guidewire as one can be very useful (Video 3, https://bit.ly/3jPF7aj and **Figure 14**). If the loop, during the crossing, becomes too large, it means that most certainly, a perforation has occurred. In these situations, the guidewire should be retracted and an another subintimal track should be pursued.

5.2.7 Retrograde access

When the antegrade approach is not successful, a retrograde puncture may be required. Retrograde puncture of the popliteal artery is usually not a big issue. However, at below-the-knee level, since arteries are quite small and fragile and

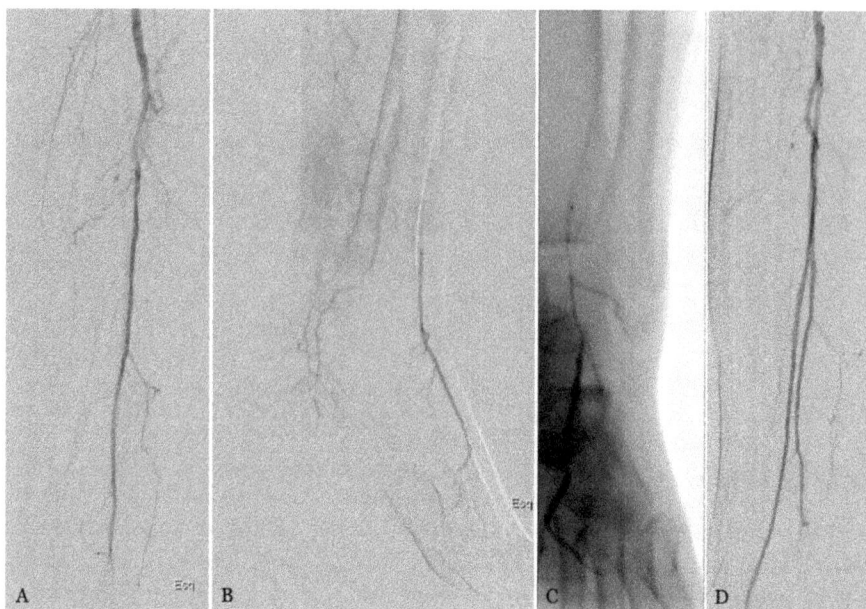

Figure 14.
A, B—Initial angiogram showing a long occlusion of the anterior tibial artery. C—Confirmation that the true lumen has been reached after a subintimal crossing of the occlusion (Video 3, https://bit.ly/3jPF7aj). D—Final result.

frequently the tibial or peroneal artery to be punctured is the unique artery to the foot, extreme care must be the rule. As so, after having performed the puncture with a 21G needle (either guided by ultrasound or by X-ray), a guidewire is to be engaged inside the artery. To avoid additional injury to the artery, the devices introduced in it should be kept at the strict minimum. That why usually it is most preferable to initially advance only the guidewire without any catheter or sheath (**Figure 15**). Therefore, the guidewire to be chosen needs to have a hydrophilic stiff body due to the lack of a sheath, the relevance of having adequate torqueability to guide the tip and to perform the snaring of the guidewire, and a potential need for an additional catheter if the guidewire does not reach the true lumen or the same subintimal track made anterogradely. A 0.018″ diameter guidewire is probably the best option as it is still a delicate guidewire, but with more support than a 0.014″ guidewire. The tip should be soft and most probably hydrophilic to track easily the punctured vessel retrogradely. As no sheath should usually be introduced, hard push on the guidewire can lead to irreversible kinking of its body, which can jeopardize the intervention.

5.2.8 Pedal plantar loop technique

This technique consists in creating a loop with the guidewire from the anterior tibial artery to the posterior tibial artery, or the reverse, through the foot vessels [8, 9]. The most common pathway is through dorsalis pedis artery, deep plantar artery, deep plantar arterial arch, lateral plantar artery, and posterior tibial artery. Indications for this technique are similar to the retrograde access. However, it can be performed when no distal vessels are available for puncture, being also less invasive. Moreover, this technique can improve the outflow for tibial arteries.

However, complications related to foot vessels manipulation can precipitate a serious worsening of the ischemic condition. Taking this into account, the guidewire to be chosen to this technique needs to have a soft hydrophilic tip to easily

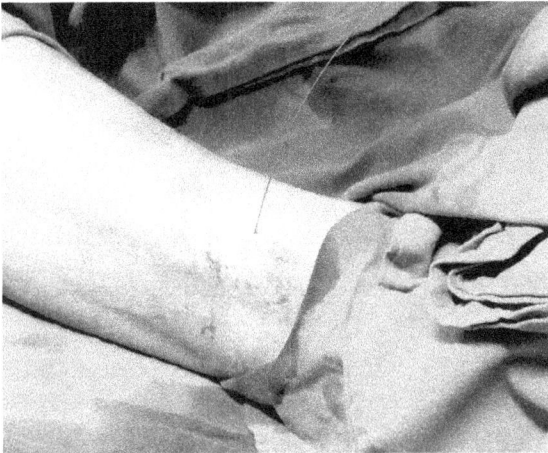

Figure 15.
After a retrograde puncture of the peroneal artery, a guidewire was inserted in it lumen, without any sheath or catheter.

track through tortuous foots vessels without damaging them. The body should also have reduced stiffness to track across the created loop, that's why usually a 0.014″ guidewire is preferred.

6. Potential guidewire-related complications

The manipulation with a guidewire of smaller vessels such as the tibial and foot arteries can precipitate vasospasm. This can be quite common in young patients or in vessels with no calcification. It is very relevant to be able to recognize it and consequently avoid the confusion with atherosclerotic stenoses and perform angioplasty on those arteries, which can lead to dissection or even rupture (**Figure 16**). Several drugs can be administered intra-arterially to solve the issue. Agents commonly used for this purpose are nitroglycerin, verapamil, or papaverine. The dose to be injected should consider the blood pressure of the patient. The hemodynamic status of the patient should also be closely checked after the administration. They ideally should be given selectively through a diagnostic catheter to the target vessel. The guidewire can be gently withdrawn to a more proximal segment of the vessel, but without losing the ostium and consequently the access to the vessel.

A perforation or an arteriovenous fistula that occurs while attempting to cross a chronic total occlusion is rarely of any clinical significance as it will almost constantly closes within few minutes when only a guidewire or a low-profile catheter has passed extraluminally [10] (**Figures 17** and **18**). Thus, one should be sure to be inside the vessel before inflating a balloon. Removing the devices to above the proximal cap of the chronic total occlusion and reattempting to cross the lesion from the top, may allow successful path and aid in solving the perforation or the arteriovenous fistula. When those complications do not auto-resolve, external compression guided by angiography or temporary vessel occlusion with a balloon can be attempted. Sometimes a covered stent may be needed. In very rare situations, coil embolization must be envisaged.

An unintended wall dissection or perforation of an intact vessel distally after having crossed the target lesion can be quite challenging to solve and can threaten the success of the procedure or even worsen the ischemic condition of the patient.

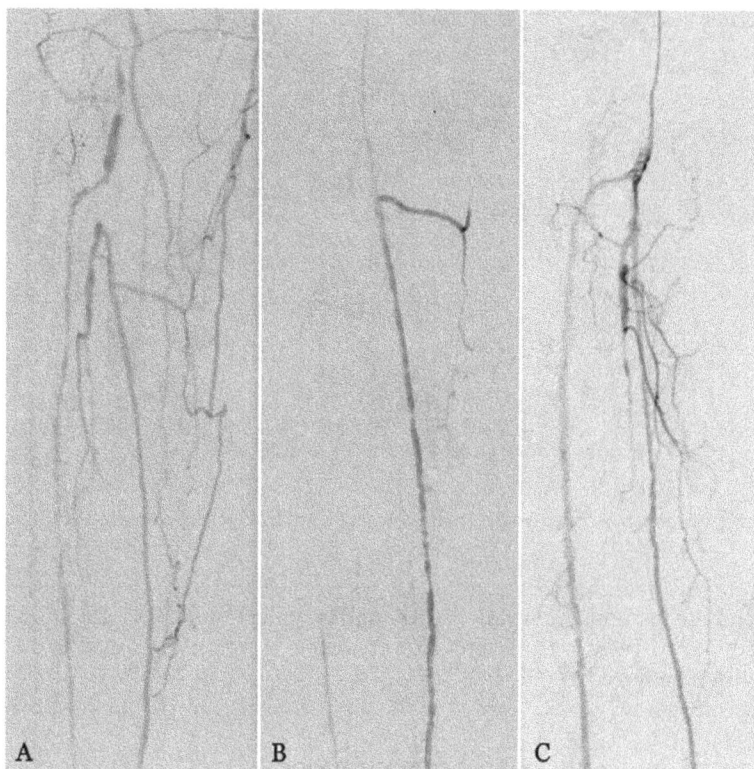

Figure 16.
A—Initial angiogram showing an occlusion of the tibioperoneal trunk and a quite healthy posterior tibial artery. B—After having crossed the occlusion, a 0.018" guidewire was advanced inside the posterior tibial artery causing diffuse spasm of the artery (string of beads appearance). C—Few minutes after having selectively administrated 200 μg of nitroglycerin, the posterior tibial artery is widely open again.

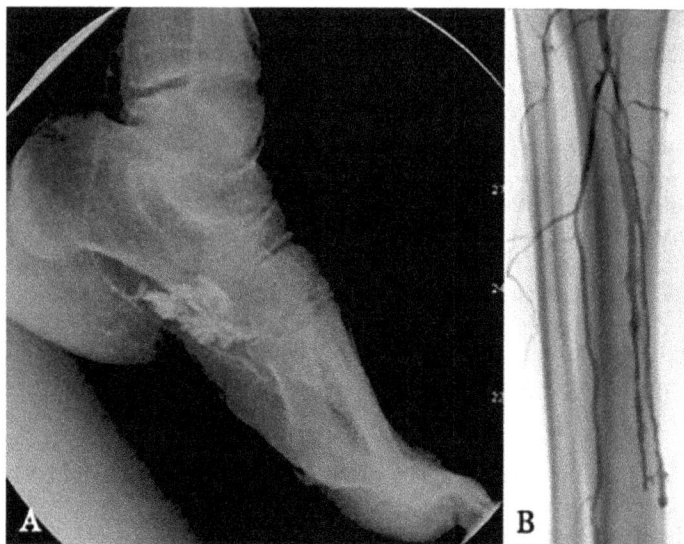

Figure 17.
A—Perforation of the lateral plantar artery; extraluminal contrast is easily noticed. B—Peroneal arteriovenous fistula. Adapted from [7].

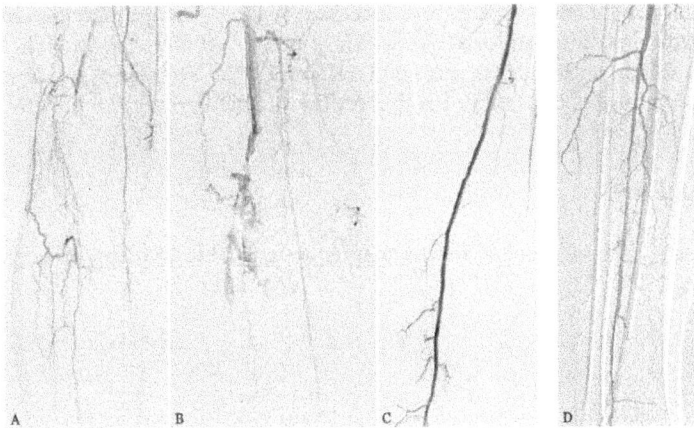

Figure 18.
A—Occlusion of the popliteal artery, tibio-peroneal trunk, and proximal segment of peroneal artery. B—Perforation occurred while trying to cross the occlusion through the initial antegrade approach. C & D—Final result after a retrograde puncture of the peroneal artery and successful crossing of the occlusion.

Therefore, the most relevant concerning this issue is to adopt correct guidewire choices and strategies to avoid it.

7. Future perspectives

X-ray fluoroscopy is still the gold standard imaging technique for the vast majority of endovascular procedures currently performed. Therefore, most of the endovascular devices, guidewires included, are designed to optimally perform under X-ray. However, its inherent ionizing radiation leads to safety concerns not only to the healthcare professionals, but also to the patients. As a result, recent advancements have been made toward magnetic resonance guided endovascular interventions [11]. Magnetic resonance imaging is a noninvasive, radiation-free imaging technique that can provide not only morphologic but also functional information (e.g., blood flow, tissue oxygenation, diffusion, or perfusion), which can potentially influence decisions during a procedure [11]. Yet, magnetic resonance guided interventions face a major challenge due to the presence of a large magnetic field, which limits the utilization of the currently available materials, including guidewires. Despite these challenges, significant progress has been recently made in the development of biocompatible, magnetic resonance safe, and visible interventional devices [11]. The guidewires presently used in the endovascular field have a long metallic core. In a magnetic resonance environment, it can create artifacts and can also induce thermal injury. As a result, new dedicated guidewires have been designed with the metallic core replaced by polymers reinforced by glass fibers or fiber composites. Those guidewires demonstrated to have improved stiffness and kink resistance [11]. Further research and development regarding magnetic resonance compatible devices and magnetic resonance imaging techniques will probably lead to a shift in the future standards of endovascular procedures.

8. Conclusions

Guidewires are the cornerstone of any endovascular revascularization. Therefore, a correct knowledge of the engineering aspects of wire technology can be the difference between failure and success as it allows an adequate guidewire choice in any situation and for each specific crossing technique. A vascular interventionist should subsequently master a relatively small number of guidewires to be able to fully translate in practice his theoretical knowledge on guidewire design.

Video materials

Video materials referenced in this chapter are available at: https://bit.ly/3jPF7aj.

Author details

Daniel Brandão[1,2]

1 Angiology and Vascular Surgery Department, Vila Nova de Gaia/Espinho Hospital Center, Portugal

2 Angiology and Vascular Surgery Unit, Faculty of Medicine of the University of Porto, Portugal

*Address all correspondence to: jdanielbrandao@gmail.com

IntechOpen

References

[1] Harrison GJ, How TV, Vallabhaneni SR, Brennan JA, Fisher RK, Naik JB, et al. Guidewire stiffness: What's in a name? Journal of Endovascular Therapy. 2011;**18**(6):797-801

[2] Lorenzoni R, Ferraresi R, Manzi M, Roffi M. Guidewires for lower extremity artery angioplasty: A review. EuroIntervention. 2015;**11**(7):799-807

[3] Lanzer P. Textbook of Catheter-Based Cardiovascular Interventions: A Knowledge-Based Approach. 2nd ed. Cham: Springer International Publishing; 2018

[4] Buller C. Coronary guidewires for chronic total occlusion procedures: Function and design. Interventional Cardiology. 2013;**5**(5):533-540

[5] Stone GW, Kandzari DE, Mehran R, Colombo A, Schwartz RS, Bailey S, et al. Percutaneous recanalization of chronically occluded coronary arteries: A consensus document: Part I. Circulation. 2005;**112**(15):2364-2372

[6] Godino C, Sharp AS, Carlino M, Colombo A. Crossing CTOs-the tips, tricks, and specialist kit that can mean the difference between success and failure. Catheterization and Cardiovascular Interventions. 2009;**74**(7):1019-1046

[7] Forbes T. Angioplasty, Various Techniques and Challenges in Treatment of Congenital and Acquired Vascular Stenoses. London: InTech; 2012

[8] Fusaro M, Dalla Paola L, Biondi-Zoccai G. Pedal-plantar loop technique for a challenging below-the-knee chronic total occlusion: A novel approach to percutaneous revascularization in critical lower limb ischemia. The Journal of Invasive Cardiology. 2007;**19**(2):E34-E37

[9] Manzi M, Fusaro M, Ceccacci T, Erente G, Dalla Paola L, Brocco E. Clinical results of below-the knee intervention using pedal-plantar loop technique for the revascularization of foot arteries. The Journal of Cardiovascular Surgery. 2009;**50**(3):331-337

[10] Lyden SP. Techniques and outcomes for endovascular treatment in the tibial arteries. Journal of Vascular Surgery. 2009;**50**(5):1219-1223

[11] Abdelaziz MEMK, Tian L, Hamady M, Yang G-Z, Temelkuran B. X-ray to MR: The progress of flexible instruments for endovascular navigation. Progress in Biomedical Engineering. 2021;**3**(3):032004

Chapter 5

Revascularization Strategies in Liver Transplantation

Flavia H. Feier, Melina U. Melere, Alex Horbe and Antonio N. Kalil

Abstract

Vascular complications following liver transplantation chan jeopardize the liver graft and recipient survival. Aggressive strategies to diagnose and treat these complications may avoid patient and graft loss. With the evolving knowledge and novel therapies, less invasive strategies are gaining importance in the treatment of post liver transplant vascular complications. Portal, hepatic, and arterial thrombosis may be managed with systemic therapies, endovascular approaches, surgical and lastly with retransplantation. The timing between the diagnosis and the directed treatment is paramount for the success. Revascularization by means of interventional radiology plays an important role in the resolution and long-term patency of arterial and venous complications. This chapter will lead the reader into the most up-to-date treatments of post liver transplant vascular complications.

Keywords: hepatic artery thrombosis, portal thrombosis, heparin, alteplase

1. Introduction

Liver transplantation (LT) is the last resource for patients with end-stage liver failure. Currently, the excellent posttransplant survival rates shift the attention to improved patient care, quality of life, and diminishing posttransplant complications. LT can be performed with deceased donors or living donors. Also, the liver can be implanted as the hole organ, as in orthotopic liver transplantation (OLT) (**Figure 1**), or partial liver (left lobe, right lobe, left lateral segment) (**Figure 2**). Technical variant grafts include partial liver grafts from living donors, split liver, and reduced grafts and have historically been associated with higher risk of posttransplant vascular complications. The indications for LT and the techniques vary according to the age of the recipient, but basically involve a total liver resection with a graft implantation that requires three vascular anastomosis [hepatic vein (HV), portal vein (PV), and hepatic artery (HA)], and a biliary anastomosis. Each of the vascular anastomosis has a potential to suffer thrombosis and/or stenosis. The early diagnosis and intervention will determine the graft and patient survival, since any one of these may be fatal [1, 2].

In the following paragraphs, a detailed review of the pathogenesis of each vascular complication and current available treatment options will be presented.

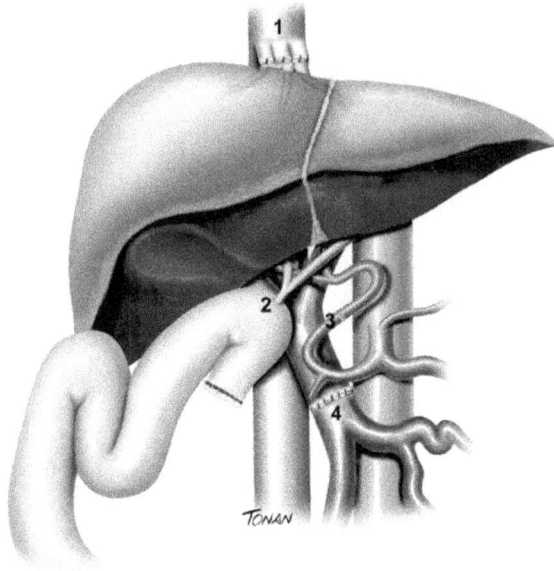

Figure 1.
Whole-liver transplant with related surgical anastomosis sites. 1= hepatic vein anastomosis using the recipients three hepatic veins and the common stump of the recipient hepatic veins by the piggyback technique; 2 = biliary anastomosis with choledochojejunostomy; 3 = HA reconstruction; and 4 = PV anastomosis [1].

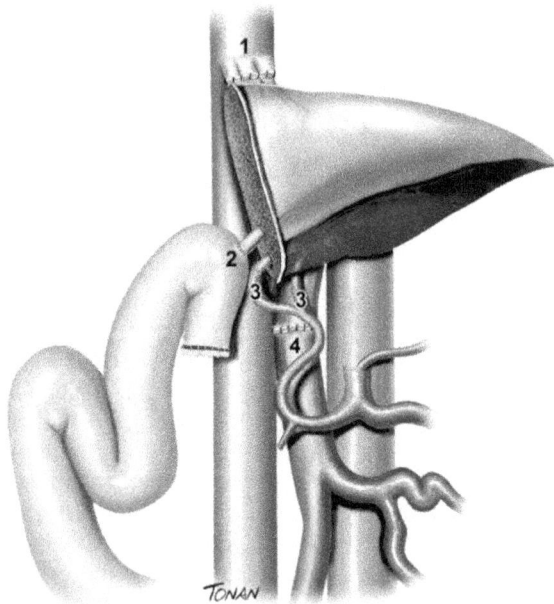

Figure 2.
Living-donor liver transplant, with left lateral liver graft with surgical anastomoses of the hepatic veins by using the piggyback technique (1), hepaticojejunostomy (2), HA reconstruction with two anastomoses (double HA technique) (3), and PV anastomosis (4) [1].

2. Hepatic vein thrombosis/stenosis

2.1 Pathogenesis and diagnosis

Hepatic vein anastomosis can be complicated by the development of stenosis and thrombosis. When venous drainage from the liver is compromised, liver parenchyma gets congested, causing impairment in the liver function, including a sluggish portal flow, and is called hepatic venous outflow obstruction (HVOO). Clinical manifestations of HVOO are nonspecific but may include abnormal liver function, hepatomegaly, ascites, pleural effusion, and lower-extremity edema. If it occurs in the immediate postoperative period, it can cause refractory graft dysfunction from liver congestion and graft loss. The mortality can be as high as 17–24% [3].

The incidence of HVOO after OLT varies from 0.5 to 9.5%. This incidence can be a little higher (3.9–16%) in living donor liver transplantation (LDLT) [4].

Routine Doppler ultrasound (DUS) performed in the immediate posttransplant period can identify signs of HVOO, such as dilated hepatic veins and dampened phasicity (pulsatility index less than 0.45) as lack of transmission of the right atrial waveform into the hepatic veins. In addition, the flow at the anastomosis often shows turbulence [5]. A computed tomography (CT) scan shows better sensitivity (97% vs. 87%) and specificity (86% vs. 68%) than DUS and allows the observation of parenchymal changes such as hypoattenuation during the portal venous phase or the delayed phase, which could suggest venous congestion [6]. The confirmation of this diagnosis is made by hepatic venography and manometry and is defined as stasis of the contrast medium from anastomotic obstruction on venography or a pressure gradient across the stenosis between the distal hepatic vein and the right atrium >5 mmHg. A pressure gradient of >5–6mmHg is widely accepted as the threshold for induction of symptoms [4].

Early complications (<30 days) are thought to be caused by technical factors such as a tight suture line, venous size match, kinking, and compression from a large graft. On the other hand, chronic (>30 days) obstructions are thought to result from fibrosis around the anastomotic site, intimal hyperplasia, twisting, or compression of the anastomosis from a hypertrophic graft [7].

Particular attention to anastomotic techniques is important such as performing a wide triangulated anastomosis, avoiding rotation of graft at the hepatocaval junction, and stabilization of the graft in an anatomical position [8]. Hepatic vein reconstruction is of particular challenge in right lobe grafts, in adult LDLT. Multiple middle hepatic vein tributaries draining the segment 5 vein (V5) are commonly found in donor hepatectomy using conventional modified right lobe grafts, leading to the performance of multiple anastomosis, including the use of vascular grafts to ensure adequate liver parenchymal drainage [4].

2.2 Revascularization and outcomes

Treatment of HVOO depends on the time of presentation and the cause (**Figure 3**). Most patients can be managed by interventional radiology (IR), performing a balloon angioplasty, with or without stent placement (**Figure 4**). During the early postoperative period, given the mechanism of HVOO, there is a high chance of restenosis if angioplasty alone is done. Stent is therefore indicated, also because balloon dilatation carries a risk of anastomosis disruption in the first days. Primary stent placement may be an effective treatment modality with an acceptable long-term patency to manage

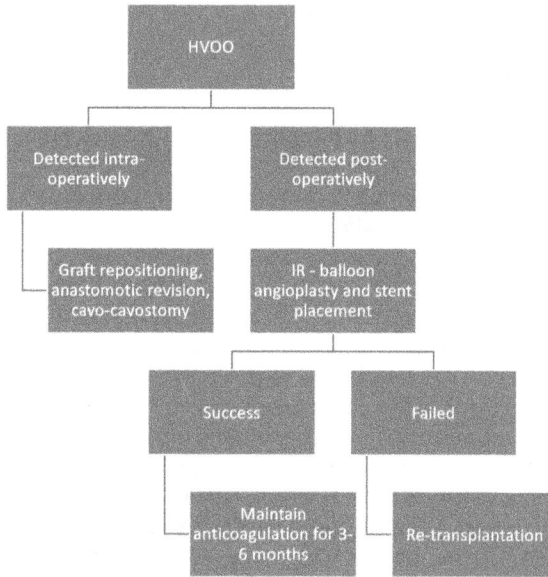

Figure 3.
Algorithm for the management of HVOO. HVOO: hepatic venous outflow obstruction; and IR: interventional radiology.

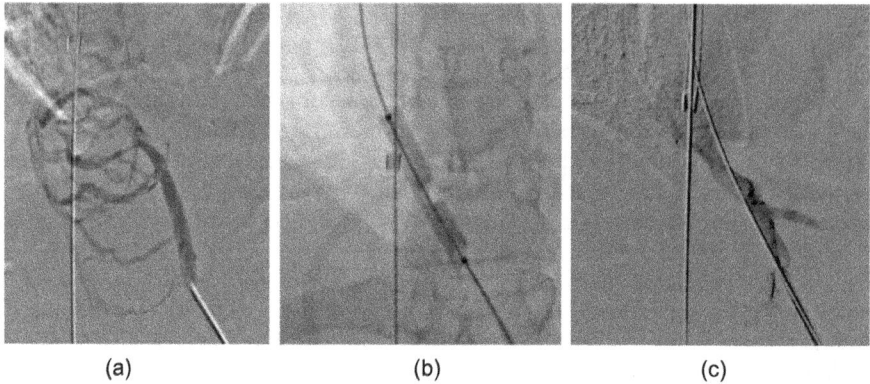

(a)   (b)   (c)

Figure 4.
Hepatic vein stenosis treated with balloon angioplasty. (a) Left hepatic vein stenosis with evidence of collateral veins. (b) Trans-hepatic access and balloon positioning in the stenosis site. (c) Final aspect after balloon dilatation with resolution of collateral veins.

early posttransplant HVOO. Jang et al reported a technical success rate of 96% and 3-year patency rate of 80% in 21 adult LDLT recipients with HVOO treated with IR [4].

Surgical options should be considered if HVOO is evident at the initial operation, which can be assessed by a transoperative DUS or in the early post-operative period. Surgery is also preferred if there is thrombosis of the hepatic veins because of the high chance of pulmonary embolism with IR treatment [5]. Retransplantation is considered as a last resource, when recanalization fails after these previous attempts.

3. Portal vein thrombosis/stenosis

3.1 Pathogenesis and diagnosis

The incidence of portal vein complications (PVCs) varies according to the recipient (children vs. adult), the LT modality (LDLT vs. OLT), and the preexistence of portal vein thrombosis (PVT). Untreated, it can lead to retransplantation, which happens in almost half of the recipients with PVT [9, 10].

The incidence of PVT after OLT can be up to 3–7%, 4% after LDLT [10], and up to 30% in children [11]. LT in children can present with additional difficulties related to portal vein reconstruction (short vascular stumps, size discrepancy between the donor's and the recipient's vascular structures, anastomotic misalignment, stenosis, anastomotic kinks, low portal flow (<7 cm/s), small portal veins (<4 mm), and use of interposition vascular grafts) that can justify the higher incidence of portal vein complications [12].

The diagnosis of PVT can be made by the detection of clinical signs (fever, abdominal pain, intractable ascites, gastrointestinal bleeding, or encephalopathy) and/or laboratory abnormalities (elevated liver enzymes, elevated ammonia levels, and/or thrombocytopenia), or detected during routine posttransplant DUS examination. Some signs present in DUS can indicate a portal vein complication: decreased or absent PV blood flow, acceleration of blood flow at the PV anastomosis, and postanastomotic jet flow. Any of these findings should prompt a CT scan. A decrease in more than 50% in PV diameter in CT scan is a sign of portal vein stenosis (PVS) even though recipient/donor mismatch should always be considered in cases of LDLT and pediatric recipients. PVT appears in the CT scan as the absence of visible lumen at the site of a thrombus [10–12].

PVT can be classified into four grades according to Yerdel [13]: Grade I: thrombus at main PV affecting less than 50% of the lumen with or without minimal extension into superior mesenteric vein (SMV); Grade II: thrombus at PV affecting more than 50%, including complete thrombosis, with or without minimal extension into the SMV; Grade III: complete PVT plus thrombosis extending to the proximal SMV with patent distal SMV; Grade IV: complete PVT plus complete thrombosis of the SMV (proximal and distal).

3.2 Revascularization and outcomes

Revascularization options for patients with PVT after LT will depend on the extension of the thrombosis and the time of onset/diagnosis. Surgical revision, systemic anticoagulation, catheter-based thrombolytic therapy, balloon angioplasty and stenting, portosystemic shunting compose the usual algorithm. Retransplantation remains as the last resource when everything else has failed [10].

Early complications (from 24 h to 1 week after LT) are usually associated with technical issues and tend to benefit from surgical revision (redo anastomosis, kinking, liver graft repositioning) (**Figure 5**). However, IR may play an important role as a salvage treatment when surgical revision of PV anastomoses fails. In contrast to early PVCs, late complications (>30 days), as well as grades 2–4 PVT, are associated with less favorable prognoses [11, 14].

Patients with grade 1 PVT without liver graft impairment can be treated with full heparinization [unfractioned or low-molecular-weight heparin (LMWH)] and then maintained anticoagulated with warfarin or rivaroxaban for 3–6 months.

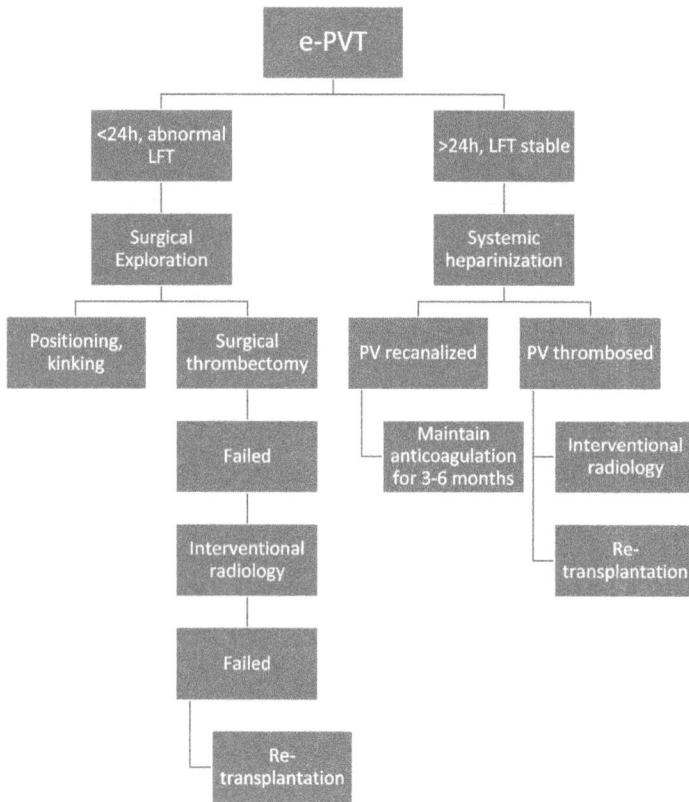

Figure 5.
Algorithm for the management of e-PVT. e-PVT: early portal vein thrombosis; LFT: liver function tests; and PV: portal vein.

IR treatment is the first choice for patients with higher grades of PVT (2–4), portal vein occlusion, failed surgical revascularization, or failed recanalization with systemic anticoagulation (**Figure 6**). Balloon angioplasty with stent placement has high rates of success and low PVT recurrence [10, 11]. The PV access can be made percutaneously (trans-hepatic or trans-splenic) or via mini-laparotomy for a direct catheterization of the portal venous system through ileo-colic or mesenteric venous branches [10].

The trans-hepatic approach is usually chosen for the first attempt; however, in patients with chronic PVT, recanalization can be difficult, precluding venoplasty [15]. The ileo-colic approach involves a mini-laparotomy, followed by a catheterization of a venous branch, introduction of a 7 F sheath, and performance of the portography. This approach has advantages in terms of the certainty of portal catheterization [10]. Another option is the trans-splenic access, which is less injurious to the transplanted liver graft (**Figure 7**) [11].

Despite the chosen access, IR protocols for PVT revascularization usually include catheterization, passage of the guidewire through the thrombosed segment, balloon angioplasty, and stent placement (**Figure 7**). A thrombolysis may be performed in order to facilitate the aspiration of the thrombus. The catheter is placed inside the thrombus and the thrombolytic agent infused. If the first treatment is considered ineffective, the catheter may be left and a continuous infusion of the thrombolytic agent maintained, from a period of 10 days to 30 days [10]. Patients are left anti-coagulated after the procedure, at least for 3 months. Sanada et al. recommended

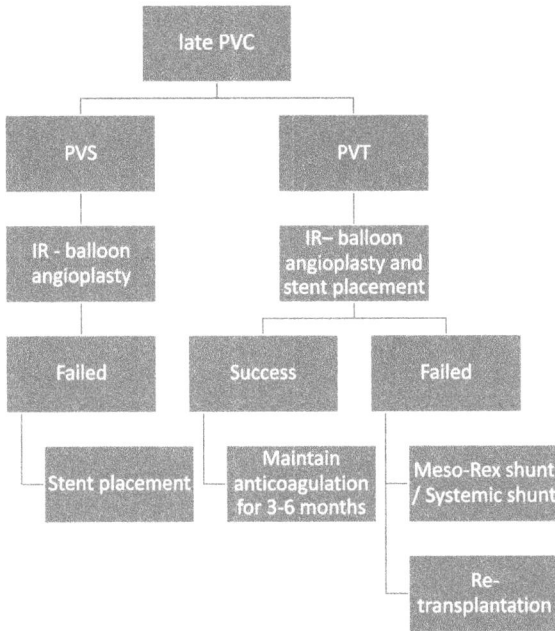

Figure 6.
Algorithm for the management of late PVC. PVC: portal vein complication; PVS: portal vein stenosis; PVT: portal vein thrombosis; and IR: interventional radiology.

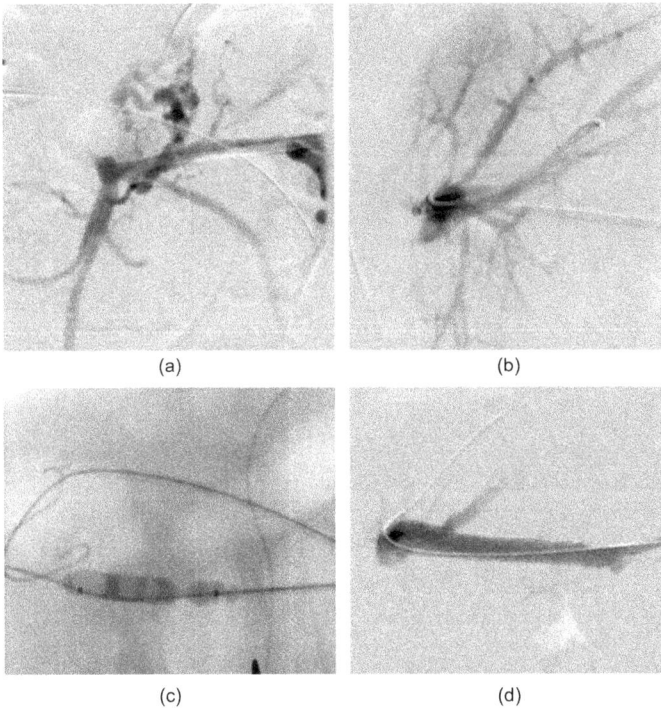

Figure 7.
Portal vein thrombosis treated with balloon angioplasty and stent. (a) Trans-splenic access and portography; (b) Passage of the guidewire through the site of thrombosis; (c) Balloon dilatation; and (d) Final aspect after stent positioning.

the use of a three-agent anticoagulant therapy that combines low-molecular-weight heparin, warfarin, and aspirin for 3 months following balloon dilation for portal vein stenosis (PVS) in pediatric liver transplantation. Recurrence of PVS reduced from 55.6 to 0% in the long-term follow-up [16].

High rate of technical success can be achieved, and recent studies focus on LDLT. In adults, a rate of 80% was achieved with long-term patency in approximately 50–60% of cases [10]. Cavalcante et al reported on pediatric LDLT recipients with chronic PVT who underwent IR with stent placement using a trans-mesenteric approach. The technical success was of 78.6%; and 31.8% developed restenosis/thrombosis and attempted a new dilatation via transhepatic access. Most of the patients (78.5%) had less than 1 year of PVT, with an 81.8% technical success rate in this group, compared with a rate of 66.7% in patients with more than 1 year of PVT [11].

In cases of PVS, balloon angioplasty is considered the first line of treatment and has produced highly successful results (**Figure 8**). However, 28–50% of these patients may develop recurrent stenosis. There is no minimal time one should wait to perform an angioplasty, even though some groups are concerned about the risk of rupture of the suture. Some cases of PVS induced by chronic PVT are not resolved with balloon angioplasty, because the wall flexibility induces easy expansion and reversion of the PV wall by inflation and deflation of the balloon. Stent placement benefits these cases [10].

Early detection and treatment of PVS or PVT are paramount to avoid portal vein occlusion. Occluded PV has a low success of stent placement. After 1 year of

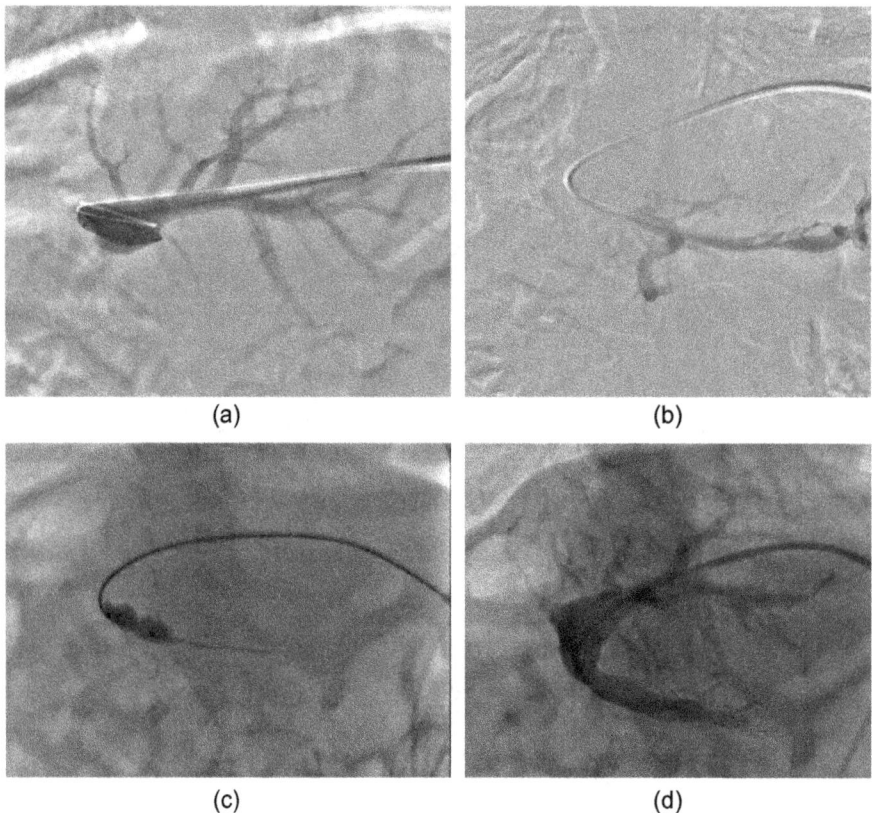

(a)   (b)

(c)   (d)

Figure 8.
Portal vein stenosis treated with balloon angioplasty. (a) Trans-hepatic access and portography; (b) Passage of the guidewire through the site of stenosis; (c) Balloon dilatation; and (d) Final aspect.

PVT, chances can be as low as 0% [17]. The treatment of a completely occluded PV is directed to the management of portal hypertension, which includes medical treatment, shunt surgery (portosystemic shunt or meso-Rex shunt), and ultimately, retransplantation (**Figure 6**) [18].

4. Hepatic artery thrombosis/stenosis

Hepatic artery complications can be classified into thrombosis and stenosis. Acute complications can be represented by early hepatic artery thrombosis (e-HAT), and chronic complications are related to late hepatic artery thrombosis (l-HAT) and hepatic artery stenosis (HAS). Revascularization strategies for these situations include surgical thrombectomy, endovascular thrombectomy, endovascular thrombolysis, systemic anticoagulation, systemic thrombolysis, and endovascular angioplasty and stent placement. The pathogenesis and best treatment modality of each type of complication will be discussed.

4.1 Early hepatic artery thrombosis

e-HAT presents early in the posttransplant course. There is lack of definition in the literature about the post-LT period in which e-HAT should be classified, some assume 14 days, some 30 days, or even as long as 100 days. It can present asymptomatically and be detected with routine posttransplant DUS, but if left untreated can lead to liver failure and retransplantation. e-HAT has been associated with high mortality rate after LT, around 33% [19].

The incidence varies according to the transplant center, the age of the recipient, the transplant modality, and surgical technique. During the initial experience, rates in children reached 42% and 12% in adult recipients. More recently, the combined reported incidence of e-HAT dropped to 4.4%, and to 1–20% in pediatric recipients. Factors such as the surgical learning curve, development of microsurgical techniques, and the routine use of magnifying lenses during arterial anastomosis are responsible for these improvements. The higher incidence reported in children can be in part explained by the smaller vessels, raising the difficulty of the anastomosis. Centers that have adopted microsurgical technique have in fact reported a low incidence of e-HAT, even with partial grafts, as is the case in LDLT [2, 20]. A study by Li et al., in the setting of adult living donor liver transplantation, reported an incidence of 1.8% of HA complications using magnifying loups instead of the microscope [21].

e-HAT can be associated to surgical technique or intraoperative positioning of the hepatic artery (kinking), and when diagnosed in the first 24h after LT, surgical reintervention to check the position of the hepatic artery, check patency, or even redo the anastomosis is the best approach (**Figure 9**). Other nonsurgical causes of e-HAT include the development of slow arterial flow during an episode of acute rejection, patient hypercoagulability, cytomegalovirus infection, and immunization status, among others. A cytomegalovirus(CMV) recipient/donor mismatch emerged as a concordant risk factor. Patients submitted to a retransplantation are also in an increased risk of e-HAT [19, 20].

Since symptoms are absent during the first hours after e-HAT, routine DUS is paramount to diagnose and immediately treat this complication. Measuring the resistive index is performed as part of the DUS evaluation. A normal resistive index value ranges between 0.60 and 0.80, and values less than 0.50 have been shown to diagnosis HAS or thrombosis with a sensitivity 60% and specificity 77%. Ultrasound can detect up to 90% of all cases of HAT, but false positives can be seen in the setting of hepatic edema, systemic hypotension, or technical aspects limiting

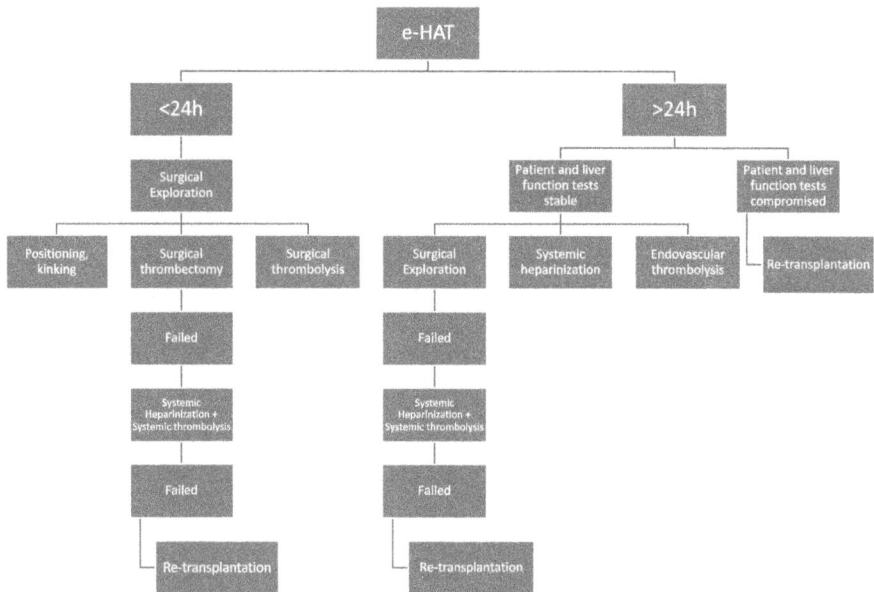

Figure 9.
Algorithm for the management of early hepatic artery thrombosis (e-HAT).

the study. CT scan has the advantage of being rapid, not operator-dependent, provides high spatial resolution of small vessels, and gives a superior anatomical overview with the aid of contrast. The combination of absent flow on DUS with confirmation on CT scan is commonly acceptable for the diagnosis of HAT. Other signs such as elevation of liver enzymes, compromise in liver function may be absent, specifically in the setting of LDLT, where the quality of the liver graft masks this alterations [2, 22, 23].

If HAT is unrecognized, the fate of the liver graft will depend on the potential for and the efficiency of developing a collateral arterial circulation and supervening infection within the compromised biliary tree. Untreated, this can progress to liver failure and death [24].

Interventions for e-HAT include urgent revascularization with thrombectomy, vascular anastomosis revision, and thrombolytic drug therapy. Traditionally, the choice was urgent retransplantation or conservative management. Most centers employ a combination of these interventions. There are no randomized controlled data to guide management. Reported studies often lack clear information about graft and patient outcomes and the selection criteria for treatment [24].

Although retransplant has been the first choice of therapy, it is associated with higher morbidity than primary transplant. Surgical options for acute HAT have traditionally included surgical revascularization and open thrombectomy. With major advancements in technology, endovascular management has emerged as a less invasive alternative treatment option.

A revascularization attempt is performed in approximately half of the cases of e-HAT, with a reported success rate of about 50% [20]. Surgical revascularization can be attempted in the first 24h after the diagnosis an e-HAT. Accerman et al performed urgent surgical revascularization in 31 children with diagnosed HAT after LT. Interventions included thrombectomy, with or without fibrinolysis, creation of a new anastomosis and conduit interposition. Success rates were reported in 61% of the cases [25]. Children are more likely than adults to have a successful outcome after early revascularization (61% of adults and 92% of children) [20, 26].

In the study of Pannaro et al., e-HAT required surgical revision in 77% patients and retransplant in 15.4%. Of the patients that required surgical revision, thrombectomy was performed in the majority and few required hepatic artery anastomotic revision. The graft salvage rate for this group was 80% [27].

In case of failed surgical revascularization, thrombolysis can still be pursued, either locally through endovascular therapy or systemically, as recently reported by our group. Systemic alteplase as a rescue therapy salvaged liver grafts in two children with e-HAT [23].

4.2 Late complications—Late HAT and HA stenosis

Late HAT manifesting months or years after surgery may be asymptomatic or have an insidious course characterized by cholangitis, relapsing fever, and bacteremia. The pathognomonic sign of HAT is the development of nonanastomotic/complex biliary stricture, most commonly at the hilum. The formation of bile casts and duct ischemia predispose the patient to recurrent cholangitis and obstructions with the development of biliary abscesses and liver infarction [2, 20, 28].

Some patients presenting l-HAT develop a neovascularized liver. Even though these patients are prone to develop biliary complications, they are treated with repeated bile duct drainage procedures (endoscopic and/or radiological), and the graft salvage rate can reach 100% [27]. Factors influencing the likelihood of spontaneous, effective collateral formation are poorly understood but include the site of the arterial thrombosis (closer to the hilum), the graft type (split/reduced grafts), Roux-en-Y hepaticojejunostomy, multiple arteries, and the timing after LT [24].

HAS is an insidious vascular complication occurring after LT. The most common complication seen in patients with HAS is biliary strictures. HAS usually occurs at or near the anastomosis site as a result of operative technique. The reported HAS rate after LT ranges from 5 to 11% [21].

HAS can be suspected when DUS presents a tardus parvus waveform (defined as a waveform with a resistive index < 0.5 and a systolic acceleration time <0.08 seconds), but has a low positive predictive value and a high false-positive rate. CT scan is indicated to confirm the diagnosis, and arteriography can be used both as a diagnostic and a treatment option [24]. Treatment options for HAS shifted from surgical reintervention to IR balloon angioplasty, with or without stent placement (**Figure 10**) [27].

Patients treated with a transluminal radiological intervention can expect a patency rate >90% within 5 years. Repeat interventions may be performed in case of HAS recurrence. Angioplasty is useful in treatment of first-time stenosis, with stenting reserved for resistant stenosis [29].

4.3 Endovascular revascularization

HAT has been reported to be successfully treated with multiple endovascular techniques, including transcatheter intra-arterial thrombolysis (IAT), percutaneous transluminal angioplasty (PTA), stenting, or a combination of these [29]. Selective thrombolysis via the hepatic artery, IAT, has several advantages such as small thrombolytic dose, high localized concentration, and little influence on systemic coagulation. It is thought to be safe and effective if the infusion catheter is placed inside the thrombus. Despite its local effect, hemorrhage is the most common complication of IAT.

Urokinase (UK) and alteplase (t-PA) are the most common thrombolytic agents used, with no documented advantage of one over the other. Thrombolytic agents (plasminogen activators) convert plasminogen into plasmin, which further cleaves the fibrin strands within the thrombus, leading to clot dissolution. t-PA is a more

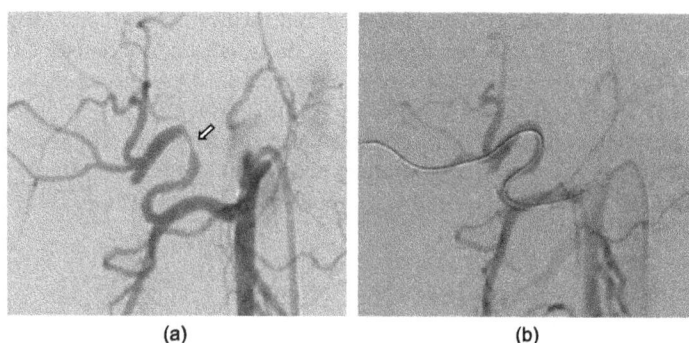

(a)　　　　　　　　　　　　　(b)

Figure 10.
Hepatic artery stenosis treated with balloon angioplasty. (a) Arteriography demonstrating the hepatic artery originating from the superior mesenteric artery and the stenosis (arrow); and (b) Final aspect after balloon dilatation.

potent activator of plasminogen and has higher affinity for fibrin within the clot. Thrombolytic agents can be infused in spaced doses [19] or continuously [30]. The lowest effective dosage and duration have not yet been determined. Dosages can vary from 1 to 3 mg (t-PA) or from 50,000 to 250,000 IU (UK) [31]. Continuous infusion can be maintained for 2–4 days with different dosing regimens, using up to 9 million units of UK [32]. Intra-arterial thrombolysis should be terminated if there is residual thrombus or persistent HAT after 36–48 h of thrombolytic therapy [33]. The estimated success rate of thrombolysis is of 68% [19].

Careful monitoring of coagulation profile and clinical symptoms is necessary during thrombolysis treatment. Fibrinogen levels should be kept above 100 mg/dl [34]; however, there is no evidence to support that fibrinogen levels are predictive of adverse bleeding; as hemorrhagic complications can also occur with values above 100 mg/dl. If adverse bleeding occurs, thrombolytic agent should be immediately terminated, and any other cause for bleeding should be addressed.

IAT can reveal other reasons for HAT, including kinking, anastomotic stenosis, or stricture, which if left untreated can lead to rethrombosis. The combined use of thrombolysis with PTA and/or stenting has been shown to have better patency and survival rates than thrombolysis alone. Angioplasty is useful in treatment of first-time stenosis, with stenting reserved for resistant stenosis [35].

4.4 Systemic thrombolysis

Medical management without surgical or endovascular intervention has yet to be confirmed as an effective treatment option for HAT. Our group recently published the successful outcome with the multimodal treatment for e-HAT after pediatric LT. Two children were successfully rescued with systemic t-PA and heparinization [23].

Posttransplant anticoagulation, even with LMWH as part of the protocol, has been shown to reduce the incidence of HAT, but does not lead to resolution (31, 32). Our posttransplant protocol includes prophylactic heparin when TTPA < 2.5 times control, and aspirin 3mg/kg when the patient resumes oral intake and platelets are >100.000. DUS is performed during the LT, in the first 24h after the transplant, and subsequently according to clinical judgment.

Systemic heparinization can salvage a liver graft after HAT if the patient has a neovascularized liver or if there is HA recanalization, which occurs less frequently. The complete understanding of how systemic heparinization or systemic thrombolysis can actually prevent retransplantation is still under debate [23, 27]. However, it is a valuable salvage therapy for these patients, and one should not hesitate in administering even if the patients go to a retransplant waiting list.

5. Conclusions

Posttransplant vascular complications jeopardize the liver graft and can impact on graft and patient survival. An impeccable surgical technique, along with close posttransplant surveillance to ensure an early diagnosis and prompt treatment, will enhance the chances to avoid retransplantation. It was not until recently that IR and thrombolysis have replaced retransplantation as the first treatment choice. Complications occurring <24 h after the LT are still best managed with surgical revision, because technical issues are usually responsible and can be addressed. Later occurring complications, however, are best managed nonoperatively, with high success rates for current therapies. Retransplantation is reserved as last resource when previous attempts have failed or when the liver grafts are already beyond salvation.

Acknowledgements

This article was funded by Teaching and Research Institute of Hospital Santa Casa de Porto Alegre, Porto Alegre, Brazil.

Author details

Flavia H. Feier*, Melina U. Melere, Alex Horbe and Antonio N. Kalil
Liver Transplantation Unit and Radiology Interventional Unit, Santa Casa de
Misericordia de Porto Alegre, Universidade Federal de Ciências da Saúde de Porto
Alegre, Porto Alegre, Brazil

*Address all correspondence to: flavia.feier@gmail.com

IntechOpen

References

[1] Horvat N, Marcelino ASZ, Horvat JV, Yamanari TR, Batista Araújo-Filho JA, Panizza P, et al. Pediatric liver transplant: Techniques and complications. Radiographics. 2017;**37**(6):1612-1631. DOI: 10.1148/rg.2017170022

[2] Neto JS, Fonseca EA, Vincenzi R, Pugliese R, Benavides MR, Roda K, et al. Technical choices in pediatric living donor liver transplantation: The path to reduce vascular complications and improve survival. Liver Transplantation. 2020;**26**(12):1644-1651. DOI: 10.1002/lt.25875

[3] Chu HH, Yi NJ, Kim HC, Lee KW, Suh KS, Jae HJ, et al. Longterm outcomes of stent placement for hepatic venous outflow obstruction in adult liver transplantation recipients. Liver Transplantation. 2016;**22**(11):1554-1561. DOI: 10.1002/lt.24598

[4] Jang JY, Jeon UB, Park JH, Kim TU, Lee JW, Chu CW, et al. Efficacy and patency of primary stenting for hepatic venous outflow obstruction after living donor liver transplantation. Acta Radiologica. 2017;**58**(1):34-40. DOI: 10.1177/0284185116637247

[5] Arudchelvam J, Bartlett A, McCall J, Johnston P, Gane E, Munn S. Hepatic venous outflow obstruction in piggyback liver transplantation: Single centre experience. ANZ Journal of Surgery. 2017;**87**(3):182-185. DOI: 10.1111/ans.13344

[6] Hwang HJ, Kim KW, Jeong WK, Song GW, Ko GY, Sung KB, et al. Right hepatic vein stenosis at anastomosis in patients after living donor liver transplantation: Optimal Doppler US venous pulsatility index and CT criteria— Receiver operating characteristic analysis. Radiology. 2009;**253**(2):543-551. DOI: 10.1148/radiol.2532081858

[7] Someda H, Moriyasu F, Fujimoto M, Hamato N, Nabeshima M, Nishikawa K,

et al. Vascular complications in living related liver transplantation detected with intraoperative and postoperative Doppler US. Journal of Hepatology. 1995;**22**(6):623-632. DOI: 10.1016/0168-8278(95)80218-5

[8] Krishna Kumar G, Sharif K, Mayer D, Mirza D, Foster K, Kelly D, et al. Hepatic venous outflow obstruction in paediatric liver transplantation. Pediatric Surgery International. 2010;**26**(4):423-425. DOI: 10.1007/s00383-010-2564-y

[9] Piardi T, Lhuaire M, Bruno O, Memeo R, Pessaux P, Kianmanesh R, et al. Vascular complications following liver transplantation: A literature review of advances in 2015. World Journal of Hepatology. 2016;**8**(1):36-57. DOI: 10.4254/wjh.v8.i1.36

[10] Tokunaga K, Furuta A, Isoda H, Uemoto S, Togashi K. Feasibility and mid- to long-term results of endovascular treatment for portal vein thrombosis after living-donor liver transplantation. Diagnostic and Interventional Radiology. 2021;**27**(1): 65-71. DOI: 10.5152/dir.2020.19469

[11] Cavalcante ACBS, Zurstrassen CE, Carnevale FC, Pugliese RPS, Fonseca EA, Moreira AM, et al. Long-term outcomes of transmesenteric portal vein recanalization for the treatment of chronic portal vein thrombosis after pediatric liver transplantation. American Journal of Transplantation. 2018;**18**(9):2220-2228. DOI: 10.1111/ajt.15022

[12] Neto JS, Fonseca EA, Feier FH, Pugliese R, Candido HL, Benavides MR, et al. Analysis of factors associated with portal vein thrombosis in pediatric living donor liver transplant recipients. Liver Transplantation. 2014;**20**(10):1157-1167. DOI: 10.1002/lt.23934

[13] Yerdel MA, Gunson B, Mirza D, Karayalçin K, Olliff S, Buckels J, et al.

Portal vein thrombosis in adults undergoing liver transplantation: Risk factors, screening, management, and outcome. Transplantation. 2000;**69**(9): 1873-1881. DOI: 10.1097/00007890-200005150-00023

[14] Rizzari MD, Safwan M, Sobolic M, Kitajima T, Collins K, Yoshida A, et al. The impact of portal vein thrombosis on liver transplant outcomes: Does grade or flow rate matter? Transplantation. 2021;**105**(2):363-371. DOI: 10.1097/TP.0000000000003235

[15] Shibata T, Itoh K, Kubo T, Maetani Y, Shibata T, Togashi K, et al. Percutaneous transhepatic balloon dilation of portal venous stenosis in patients with living donor liver transplantation. Radiology. 2005;**235**(3):1078-1083. DOI: 10.1148/radiol.2353040489

[16] Sanada Y, Kawano Y, Mizuta K, Egami S, Hayashida M, Wakiya T, et al. Strategy to prevent recurrent portal vein stenosis following interventional radiology in pediatric liver transplantation. Liver Transplantation. 2010;**16**(3):332-339. DOI: 10.1002/lt.21995

[17] Cheng YF, Ou HY, Tsang LL, Yu CY, Huang TL, Chen TY, et al. Vascular stents in the management of portal venous complications in living donor liver transplantation. American Journal of Transplantation. 2010;**10**(5):1276-1283. DOI: 10.1111/j.1600-6143.2010.03076.x

[18] Sambommatsu Y, Shimata K, Ibuki S, Narita Y, Isono K, Honda M, et al. Portal vein complications after adult living donor liver transplantation: Time of onset and deformity patterns affect long-term outcomes. Liver Transplantation. 2021;**27**(6):854-865. DOI: 10.1002/lt.25977

[19] Singhal A, Stokes K, Sebastian A, Wright HI, Kohli V. Endovascular treatment of hepatic artery thrombosis following liver transplantation.

Transplant International. 2010;**23**(3): 245-256. DOI: 10.1111/j.1432-2277.2009.01037.x

[20] Bekker J, Ploem S, de Jong KP. Early hepatic artery thrombosis after liver transplantation: A systematic review of the incidence, outcome and risk factors. American Journal of Transplantation. 2009;**9**(4):746-757. DOI: 10.1111/j.1600-6143.2008.02541.x

[21] Li PC, Thorat A, Jeng LB, Yang HR, Li ML, Yeh CC, et al. Hepatic artery reconstruction in living donor liver transplantation using surgical loupes: Achieving low rate of hepatic arterial thrombosis in 741 consecutive recipients-tips and tricks to overcome the poor hepatic arterial flow. Liver Transplantation. 2017;**23**(7):887-898. DOI: 10.1002/lt.24775

[22] Banc-Husu AM, Anupindi SA, Lin HC. Resolution of hepatic artery thrombosis in 2 pediatric liver transplant patients. Journal of Pediatric Gastroenterology and Nutrition. 2016;**62**(4):546-549. DOI: 10.1097/MPG.0000000000001016

[23] Feier FH, Melere MU, Trein CS, da Silva CS, Lucchese A, Horbe A, et al. Early hepatic arterial thrombosis in liver transplantation: Systemic intravenous alteplase as a potential rescue treatment after failed surgical revascularization. Pediatric Transplantation. 2021;**25**(5): e13902. DOI: 10.1111/petr.13902

[24] Heaton ND. Hepatic artery thrombosis: Conservative management or retransplantation? Liver Transplantation. 2013;**19**(Suppl. 2): S14-S16

[25] Ackermann O, Branchereau S, Franchi-Abella S, Pariente D, Chevret L, Debray D, et al. The long-term outcome of hepatic artery thrombosis after liver transplantation in children: Role of urgent revascularization. American Journal of Transplantation.

2012;**12**(6):1496-1503. DOI: 10.1111/j.1600-6143.2011.03984.x

[26] Warnaar N, Polak WG, de Jong KP, de Boer MT, Verkade HJ, Sieders E, et al. Long-term results of urgent revascularization for hepatic artery thrombosis after pediatric liver transplantation. Liver Transplantation. 2010;**16**(7):847-855. DOI: 10.1002/lt.22063

[27] Panaro F, Gallix B, Bouyabrine H, Ramos J, Addeo P, Testa G, et al. Liver transplantation and spontaneous neovascularization after arterial thrombosis: "the neovascularized liver". Transplant International. 2011;**24**(9): 949-957. DOI: 10.1111/j.1432-2277. 2011.01293.x

[28] Grimaldi C, di Francesco F, Chiusolo F, Angelico R, Monti L, Muiesan P, et al. Aggressive prevention and preemptive management of vascular complications after pediatric liver transplantation: A major impact on graft survival and long-term outcome. Pediatric Transplantation. 2018;**22**(8): e13288

[29] Pereira K, Salsamendi J, Dalal R, Quintana D, Bhatia S, Fan J. Percutaneous endovascular therapeutic options in treating posttransplant hepatic artery thrombosis with the aim of salvaging liver allografts: Our experience. Experimental and Clinical Transplantation. 2016;**14**(5):542-550. DOI: 10.6002/ect.2015.0189

[30] Figueras J, Busquets J, Dominguez J, Sancho C, Casanovas-Taltavull T, Rafecas A, et al. Intra-arterial thrombolysis in the treatment of acute hepatic artery thrombosis after liver transplantation. Transplantation. 1995;**59**(9):1356-1357

[31] Boyvat F, Aytekin C, Karakayali H, Ozyer U, Sevmis S, Emiroğlu R, et al. Stent placement in pediatric patients with hepatic artery stenosis or

thrombosis after liver transplantation. Transplantation Proceedings. 2006;**38**(10):3656-3660. DOI: 10.1016/j.transproceed.2006.10.169

[32] Zhou J, Fan J, Wang JH, Wu ZQ, Qiu SJ, Shen YH, et al. Continuous transcatheter arterial thrombolysis for early hepatic artery thrombosis after liver transplantation. Transplantation Proceedings. 2005;**37**(10):4426-4429. DOI: 10.1016/j.transproceed.2005.10.113

[33] Saad S, Tanaka K, Inomata Y, Uemoto S, Ozaki N, Okajima H, et al. Portal vein reconstruction in pediatric liver transplantation from living donors. Annals of Surgery. 1998;**227**(2):275-281. DOI: 10.1097/00000658-199802000-00018

[34] Semba CP, Bakal CW, Calis KA, Grubbs GE, Hunter DW, Matalon TA, et al. Alteplase as an alternative to urokinase. Advisory Panel on Catheter-Directed Thrombolytic Therapy. Journal of Vascular and Interventional Radiology. 2000;**11**(3):279-287. DOI: 10.1016/s1051-0443(07)61418-3

[35] Laštovičková J, Peregrin J. Percutaneous transluminal angioplasty of hepatic artery stenosis in patients after orthotopic liver transplantation: Mid-term results. Cardiovascular and Interventional Radiology. 2011;**34**(6): 1165-1171. DOI: 10.1007/s00270-010-0082-x

The Holistic Spectrum of Thrombotic Ocular Complications: Recent Advances with Diagnosis, Prevention, and Management Guidelines

Prasanna Venkatesh Ramesh, Shruthy Vaishali Ramesh,
Prajnya Ray, Aji Kunnath Devadas, Tensingh Joshua,
Anugraha Balamurugan, Meena Kumari Ramesh
and Ramesh Rajasekaran

Abstract

Thromboembolic manifestations of the eye can vary from a trivial tributary retinal vein occlusion to a catastrophic cerebral venous sinus thrombosis. These conditions can be classified as pathologies directly affecting the eye or those causing secondary lesions due to systemic issues and can be managed accordingly. Also, recently the incidence of thrombotic phenomenon affecting multiple organs (with the eye being no exception) is estimated to be around 25% among patients hospitalized in the intensive care unit for COVID-19, even though anticoagulant treatment was administered prophylactically. In this chapter, the various patho-physiologies of the ocular thrombotic events are highlighted with a special focus on the COVID-19 induced thrombotic ocular complications. Ophthalmologists, sometimes being the first responder, have a vigilant role to play with a heightened awareness of these atypical extrapulmonary thrombotic ocular manifestations, which are not only vision-threatening; in certain instances, life-threatening too. This chapter summarizes the recent advances in ocular thrombotic diseases with focal points on the current recommendations in COVID-19 induced ocular throm-botic complications. The potential diagnostic and preventive actions such as the prophylactic role of anti-thrombotic therapy, baseline non-contrast chest computed tomography, as well as recommendations for patients with COVID-19 infection are discussed in detail.

Keywords: Thrombotic Ocular Complications, Central Retinal Vein Occlusion, Central Retinal Artery Occlusion, COVID-19 Induced Thrombotic Complications, Cerebral Venous Thrombosis, Dural Sinus Thrombosis

1. Introduction

Thromboembolic manifestations of the eye can vary from a trivial tributary retinal vein occlusion to a catastrophic cerebral venous sinus thrombosis, leading to ocular associations. These conditions can be classified as pathologies directly affecting the eye or those causing secondary lesions due to systemic issues. It is important to have an understanding and knowledge regarding the ophthalmic signs and symptoms of thromboembolic manifestations considering its systemic implications, to identify patients at risk of developing such diseases and reduce the risk of developing systemic involvement. In this chapter, the thromboembolic phenomenon and its management ranging from medical to surgical (thrombectomy) are described in detail both from an ophthalmologist and a non-ophthalmic (intensivist, emergency physician, neurologist & anesthesiologist) point of view, in managing not only the vision-threatening aspect, but also the life-threatening part of these pathologies effectively.

2. Disease spectrum

The various artery and venous thromboembolic phenomena affecting the eye are shown in **Figure 1**.

2.1 Retinal vein occlusions

2.1.1 Disease entity

Retinal vein occlusions (RVO) are a group of disorders that have an impaired venous return in common [1]. It is the second leading cause of retinal vascular blindness after diabetic retinopathy. Classification of RVO depends on the site of obstruction. If the occlusion occurs within or posterior to the optic nerve head, it is

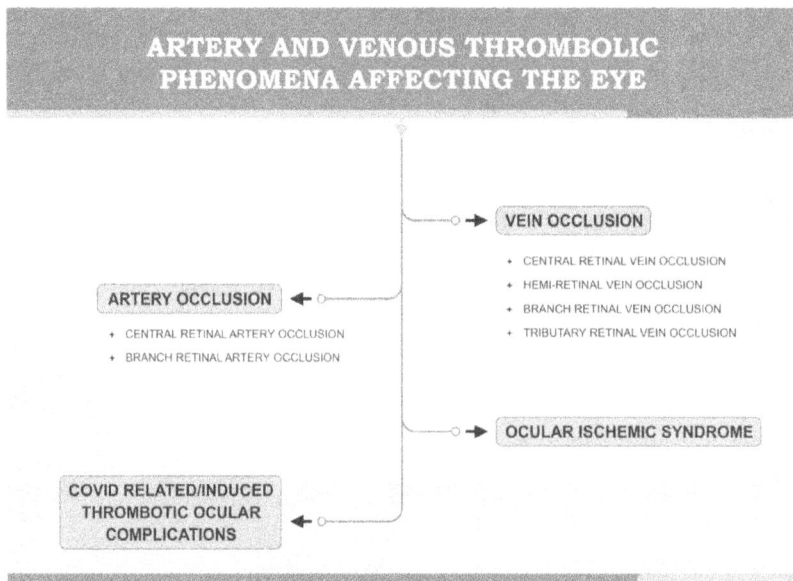

ARTERY AND VENOUS THROMBOLIC PHENOMENA AFFECTING THE EYE

VEIN OCCLUSION
+ CENTRAL RETINAL VEIN OCCLUSION
+ HEMI-RETINAL VEIN OCCLUSION
+ BRANCH RETINAL VEIN OCCLUSION
+ TRIBUTARY RETINAL VEIN OCCLUSION

ARTERY OCCLUSION
+ CENTRAL RETINAL ARTERY OCCLUSION
+ BRANCH RETINAL ARTERY OCCLUSION

OCULAR ISCHEMIC SYNDROME

COVID RELATED/INDUCED THROMBOTIC OCULAR COMPLICATIONS

Figure 1.
Various artery and venous thromboembolic phenomena affecting the eye.

termed as central retinal vein occlusion (CRVO), occlusion at the level of major bifurcation is termed as hemiretinal vein occlusion (HRVO), and occlusion within a tributary is termed as branch retinal vein occlusion (BRVO). CRVO can further be classified into ischemic CRVO and non-ischemic CRVO [2].

2.1.2 Etiopathogenesis

Majority of the RVOs are commonly associated with typical atherosclerosis, but it can be secondary to other conditions such as inflammation, vasospasm, or compressions [3]. The atherosclerotic causes include systemic arterial hypertension, arteriosclerosis, diabetes, and thrombophilia [4, 5]. BRVO commonly occurs due to venous compression at the arteriovenous crossing, whereas CRVO is most likely linked to glaucoma and sleep apnea [6, 7]. In young individuals we need to look out for uncommon associations like thrombophilia and homocystinuria [8, 9]. So RVOs is caused by three mechanisms (Videos 1, https://www.youtube.com/watch?v=JSC_E9vPnG0 and 2, https://www.youtube.com/watch?v=-wT5biKVxtE):

- Occlusion of the vein externally

- Occlusion of the vein due to degenerative inflammation of the vessel wall

- Hemodynamic disturbances [10]

According to Eye Disease Case–Control Study, CRVO is associated with the following risk factors:

- Systemic arterial hypertension

- Open-angle glaucoma

- Diabetes mellitus

- Hyperlipidemia [11]

According to Eye Disease Case–Control Study, BRVO is associated with the following risk factors:

- Increasing age

- Systemic arterial hypertension

- Smoking

- Glaucoma [4]

2.1.3 Clinical features

Symptoms are varied depending on the region involved. Sometimes symptoms of RVO can be subtle, especially if the severity is mild or the area affected does not involve the macula [12]. In cases of non-ischemic CRVO, the patient is usually asymptomatic and may be detected as an incidental finding on routine examination, revealing mild retinal hemorrhages and retinal venous stasis. The patient might have experienced amaurosis fugax before developing a constant blur in certain cases.

2.1.3.1 Clinical features of ischemic CRVO

In ischemic CRVO, patient complaints unilateral loss of vision and experiences marked loss of visual acuity, frequently noted on waking up in the morning. Visual acuity is usually counting fingers or worse, with a poor visual prognosis considering the macular ischemia. Relative afferent pupillary defect (RAPD) is typically seen here [13]. Sometimes patients would have ignored or not noticed a prior reduction in vision and might present with a painful eye, following the development of neovascular glaucoma (NVG) (**Figure 2a**). This is also known as hundred-day glaucoma [14, 15]. Such cases would present with raised intraocular pressure, corneal edema, and neovascularization of the iris (**Figure 3**). Routine gonioscopy is mandatory to check for angle neovascularization. Fundus evaluation (**Figure 4a** and **b**) will show severe tortuosity and dilatation of all the branches of the central retinal vein with extensive dot-blot and flame-shaped hemorrhages. Early signs include severe optic disc hyperemia, optic disc edema and retinal edema, especially macular edema. Cotton wool spots are typically seen here, more than in non-ischemic type. Here the acute signs start to resolve over 9–12 months. The macula develops chronic cystoid macular edema (CME), atrophic changes, epiretinal membrane, and retinal pigment epithelium changes in later stages. Retinal neovascularization is seen in about 5% of the eyes, leading to severe vitreous hemorrhages (**Figure 2b**) in most of the eyes. Optic disc collaterals are common and can reduce the risk of anterior and posterior segment neovascularization.

2.1.3.2 Clinical features of non-ischemic CRVO

Non-ischemic CRVO is also called venous stasis retinopathy. It is more common than the ischemic type, but one-third of these patients will progress towards ischemic CRVO. Visual acuity is better than 6/60 in majority of the cases and vision returns to near normal in about 50% of the cases. Poor vision would be seen in cases with chronic macular edema leading to secondary atrophy. The clinical features of non-ischemic CRVO are shown in **Figure 5**.

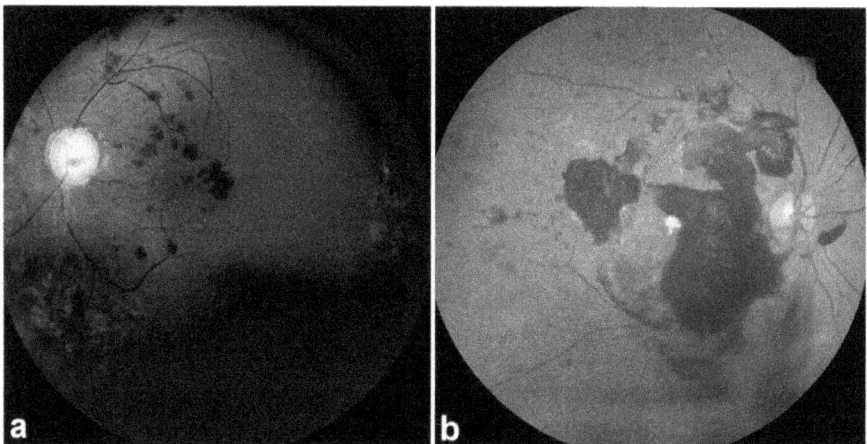

Figure 2.
(a) Fundus photograph showing total glaucomatous cupping secondary to NVG with panretinal photocoagulation LASER marks. (b) Fundus photograph showing CRVO with neovascularization elsewhere and vitreous hemorrhage.

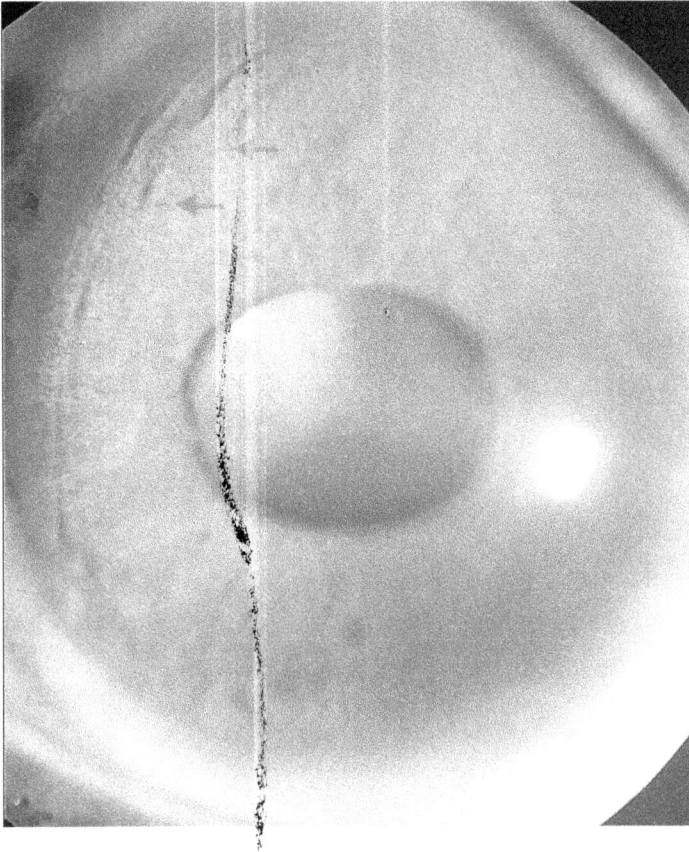

Figure 3.
Anterior segment slit lamp photograph showing neovascularization of iris (red arrows) and ectropion uveae with mid-dilated pupil.

2.1.3.3 Clinical features of BRVO

In BRVO, there is sudden unilateral painless visual loss, asymptomatic if there is no macular edema. The superotemporal quadrant (**Figure 6**) is the most commonly affected at the arteriovenous crossing point. There is dilatation and tortuosity of the affected venous segment with associated retinal hemorrhages and macular edema. Following the acute phase, resolution starts within 6–12 months with associated venous sheathing and sclerosis. Collateral vessels (**Figure 7a**) may form near the region of decreased capillary perfusion. In BRVO, it is seen between the inferior and superior vascular arcades, crossing the horizontal raphe. The presence of collaterals indicates better prognosis and care should be taken during laser to avoid hitting it. Retinal neovascularizations are more common than CRVO and are seen in about 8% of eyes.

2.1.3.4 Clinical features of macular BRVO (tributary vein occlusion)

Macular BRVO (**Figure 8**) is another variant where only the venule within the macula is occluded. Occlusion of a small macular tributary branch vein, not involving a major arcade, can be extremely subtle with minimal hemorrhage, telangiectasia or macular edema, and the correct diagnosis is frequently missed [16].

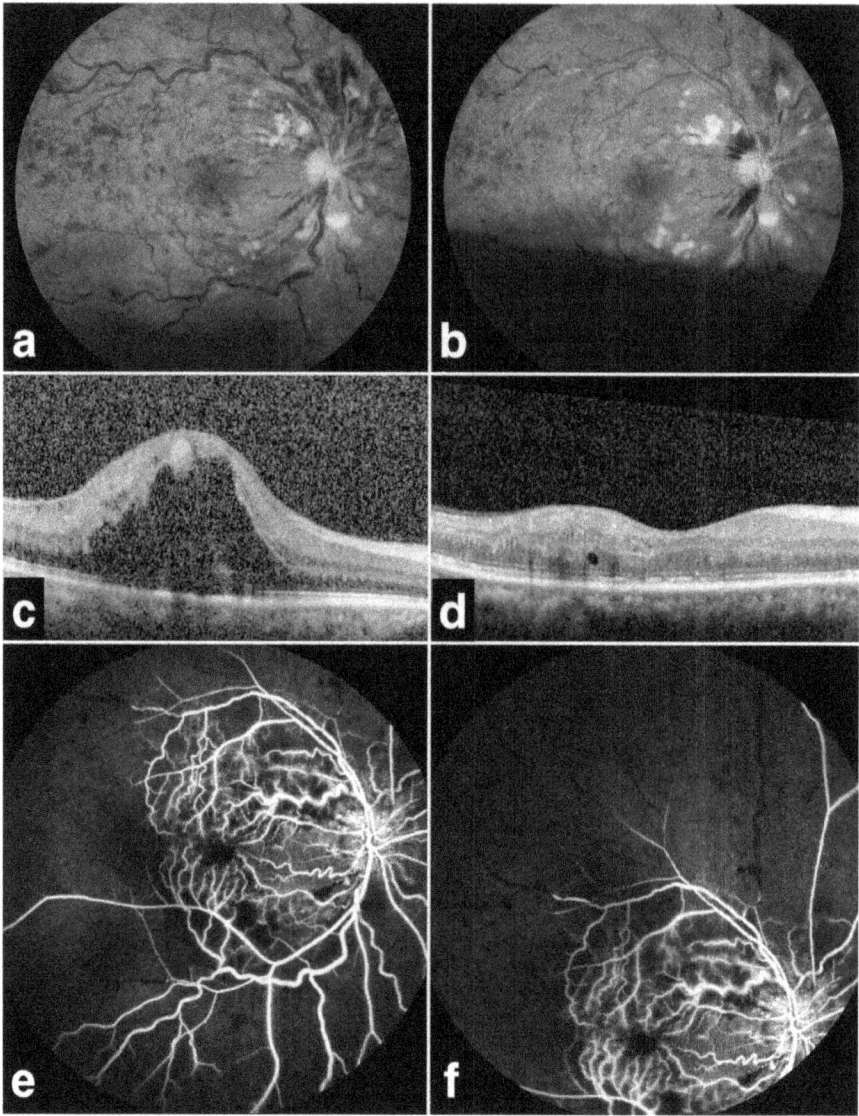

Figure 4.
(a) Fundus photograph showing ischemic CRVO with dilated and tortuous veins, several flame-shaped hemorrhages, and cotton-wool spots with disc edema. (b) Fundus photograph showing resolution of hemorrhages. (c) Optical coherence tomography (OCT) of the macula of the same case showing cystoid macular edema (CME). (d) OCT macula post anti-vascular endothelial growth factor injection showing resolution of CME. (e) Fluorescein angiography (FA) showing extensive areas of capillary nonperfusion with vessel wall staining. (f) FA showing ischemia in the peripheral zones.

2.1.3.5 Clinical features of HRVO

HRVO (**Figure 9**) is a variant of CRVO. The site of occlusion is within the optic nerve which is associated with corresponding disc edema [17]. It is less common than CRVO and BRVO. It either involves the superior or inferior branch of the central retinal vein. Signs are similar to that of CRVO, but involves only a single hemisphere.

CLINICAL FEATURES OF NON– ISCHEMIC CRVO

POOR VISUAL ACUITY

CYSTOID MACULAR EDEMA

DILATATION AND TORTUOSITY OF VEINS

RETINAL HEMORRHAGES

PATCHY OR PERI-VENULAR ISCHEMIC RETINAL WHITENING

DISC COLLATERALS

Figure 5.
Clinical features of non-ischemic CRVO.

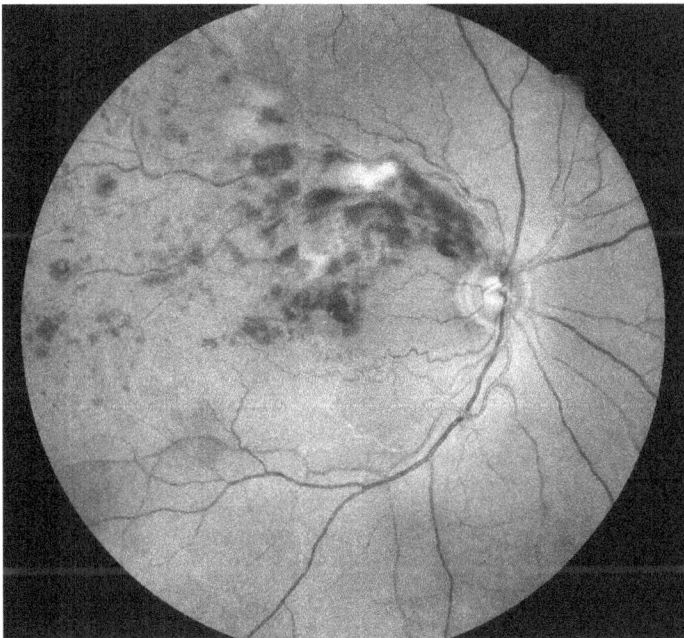

Figure 6.
Fundus photograph showing superotemporal BRVO with retinal hemorrhage, and cotton wool spots. Retinal pigment changes in the macula, with collaterals and ghost vessels in the inferotemporal quadrant.

2.1.4 Ocular investigations

Fluorescein angiography (FA) (**Figure 10**) is important to differentiate between ischemic and non-ischemic CRVO. FA will show delayed arteriovenous transit time,

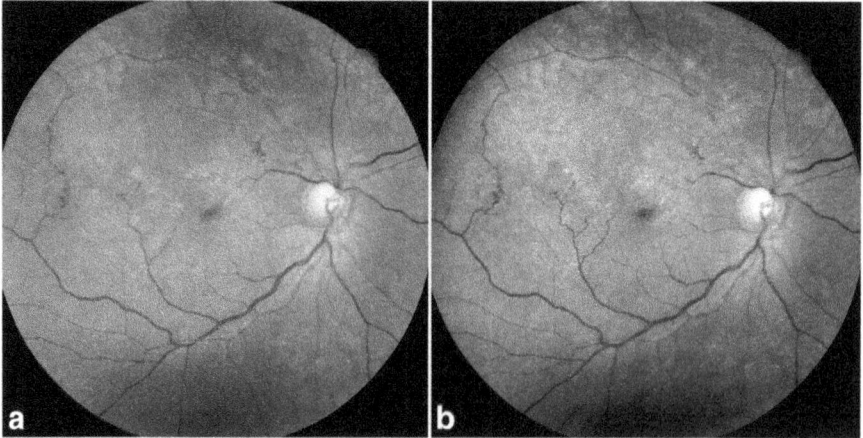

Figure 7.
(a) An old BRVO showing multiple optociliary shunts with an epiretinal membrane in the macula. (b) Fundus photo showing the same fundus after treatment with sectoral laser photocoagulation.

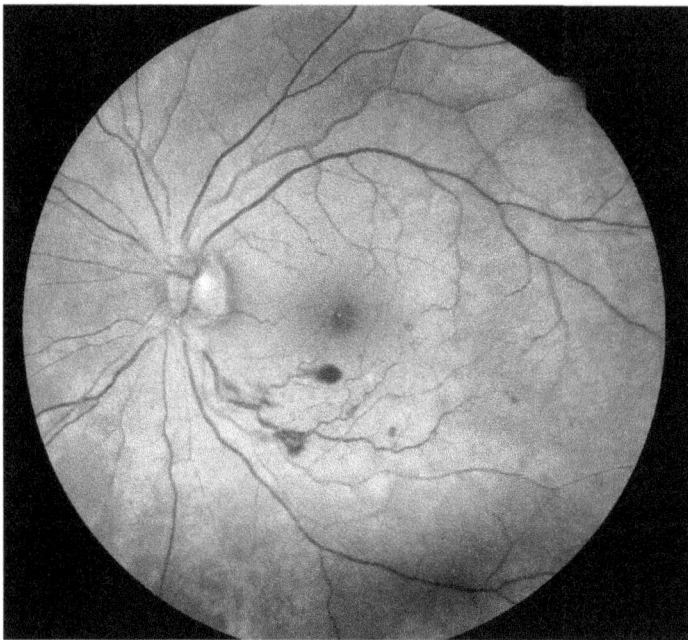

Figure 8.
Tributary vein occlusion. A venule within the macula is occluded showing few retinal hemorrhages in the involved area.

with good capillary perfusion and some late leakage in non-ischemic CRVO. In ischemic CRVO there will be extensive areas of capillary nonperfusion accompanied with vessel wall staining and leaking (**Figure 4e** and **f**). More than 10 disc areas of capillary nonperfusion are associated with an increased risk of neovascularization. As retinal hemorrhages cause blocked fluorescence, extensive hemorrhages will fail to provide us with adequate information on capillary nonperfusion areas [1, 18]. FA will also help exclude substantial macular ischemia prior to grid laser therapy.

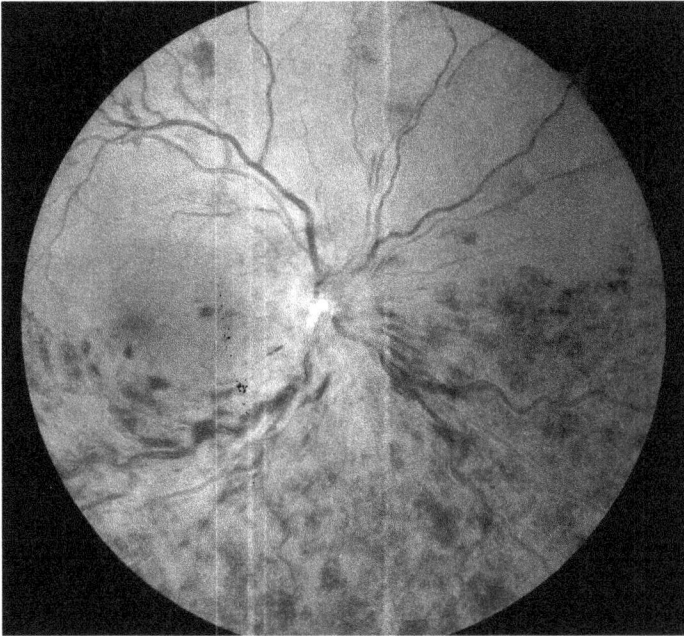

Figure 9.
Hemiretinal vein occlusion (HRVO). HRVO of the inferior branch of the central retinal vein with moderate flame-shaped hemorrhages in the inferior quadrants with associated disc edema.

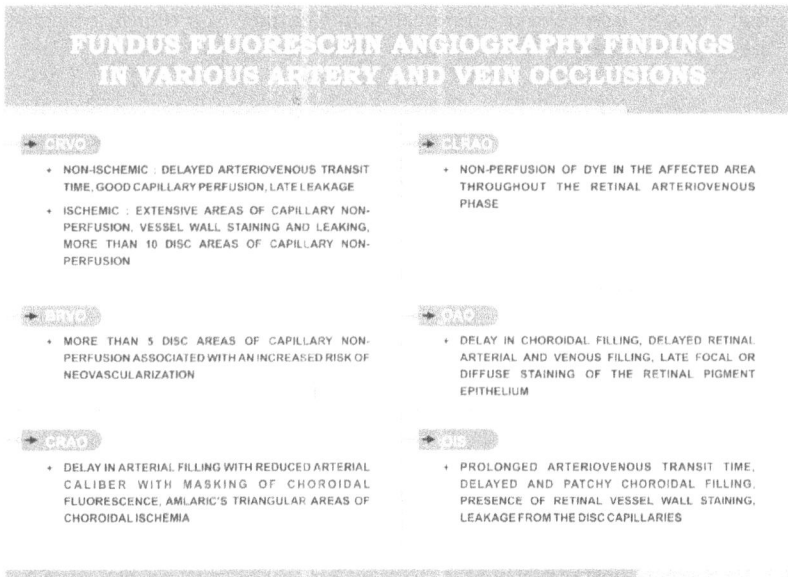

FUNDUS FLUORESCEIN ANGIOGRAPHY FINDINGS IN VARIOUS ARTERY AND VEIN OCCLUSIONS

CRVO
- NON-ISCHEMIC : DELAYED ARTERIOVENOUS TRANSIT TIME, GOOD CAPILLARY PERFUSION, LATE LEAKAGE
- ISCHEMIC : EXTENSIVE AREAS OF CAPILLARY NON-PERFUSION, VESSEL WALL STAINING AND LEAKING, MORE THAN 10 DISC AREAS OF CAPILLARY NON-PERFUSION

CLRAO
- NON-PERFUSION OF DYE IN THE AFFECTED AREA THROUGHOUT THE RETINAL ARTERIOVENOUS PHASE

BRVO
- MORE THAN 5 DISC AREAS OF CAPILLARY NON-PERFUSION ASSOCIATED WITH AN INCREASED RISK OF NEOVASCULARIZATION

OAO
- DELAY IN CHOROIDAL FILLING, DELAYED RETINAL ARTERIAL AND VENOUS FILLING, LATE FOCAL OR DIFFUSE STAINING OF THE RETINAL PIGMENT EPITHELIUM

CRAO
- DELAY IN ARTERIAL FILLING WITH REDUCED ARTERIAL CALIBER WITH MASKING OF CHOROIDAL FLUORESCENCE, AMLARIC'S TRIANGULAR AREAS OF CHOROIDAL ISCHEMIA

OIS
- PROLONGED ARTERIOVENOUS TRANSIT TIME, DELAYED AND PATCHY CHOROIDAL FILLING, PRESENCE OF RETINAL VESSEL WALL STAINING, LEAKAGE FROM THE DISC CAPILLARIES

Figure 10.
Fundus fluorescein angiographic findings in various artery, and vein occlusions.

Similarly, in BRVO more than 5 disc areas of capillary nonperfusion is associated with an increased risk of neovascularization.

OCT macula (**Figure 4c**) is used to confirm the presence of CME and quantify it, which is often mild in a non-ischemic case.

2.1.5 Systemic investigations

RVOs are multifactorial in origin and a whole host of factors acting in different combinations are the cause for an occlusion [17]. So considering this it is mandatory to do a thorough workup as shown in **Figure 11a**.

2.1.5.1 Systemic investigations in special cases of RVO

A selective series of tests need to be done in patients under the age of 50, in bilateral RVO, patients with previous thrombosis or a family history of thrombosis, and some patients in whom the above investigations are negative. The battery of investigations suggested is shown in **Figure 11b**.

2.1.6 Treatment

2.1.6.1 CRVO management

2.1.6.1.1 Intravitreal anti-vascular endothelial growth factor (VEGF) therapy

Study of Efficacy and Safety of Ranibizumab Injection in Patients with Macular Edema Secondary to Central Retinal Vein Occlusion (CRUISE) shows that 0.5 mg or 0.3 mg of monthly injections of ranibizumab were found effective in the treatment of CME [19].

Vascular Endothelial Growth Factor Trap-Eye: Investigation of Efficacy and Safety in Central Retinal Vein Occlusion (GALILEO and COPERNICUS) studies shows that monthly injections of aflibercept can be utilized for the treatment of macular edema secondary to CRVO (**Figure 4c** and **d**) [20].

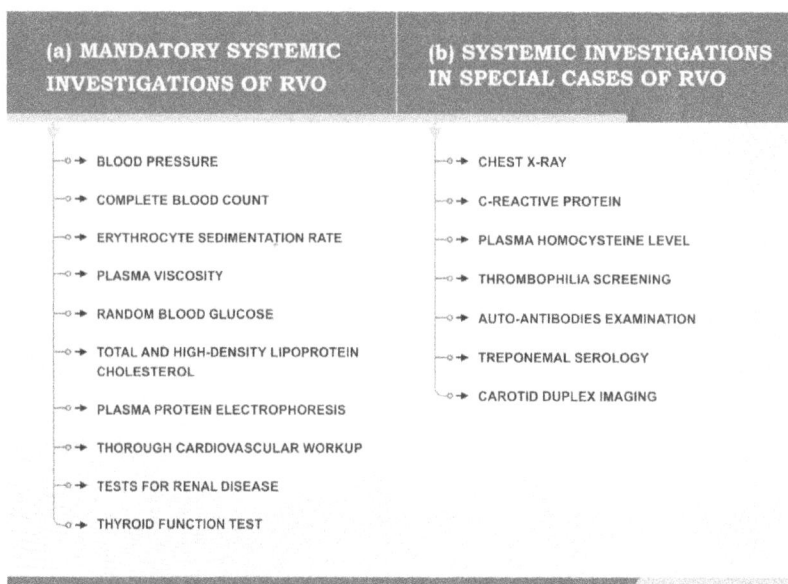

(a) MANDATORY SYSTEMIC INVESTIGATIONS OF RVO	(b) SYSTEMIC INVESTIGATIONS IN SPECIAL CASES OF RVO
BLOOD PRESSURE	CHEST X-RAY
COMPLETE BLOOD COUNT	C-REACTIVE PROTEIN
ERYTHROCYTE SEDIMENTATION RATE	PLASMA HOMOCYSTEINE LEVEL
PLASMA VISCOSITY	THROMBOPHILIA SCREENING
RANDOM BLOOD GLUCOSE	AUTO-ANTIBODIES EXAMINATION
TOTAL AND HIGH-DENSITY LIPOPROTEIN CHOLESTEROL	TREPONEMAL SEROLOGY
PLASMA PROTEIN ELECTROPHORESIS	CAROTID DUPLEX IMAGING
THOROUGH CARDIOVASCULAR WORKUP	
TESTS FOR RENAL DISEASE	
THYROID FUNCTION TEST	

Figure 11.
(a) Systemic investigations done in retinal vein occlusion cases. (b) Systemic investigations done in special cases of retinal vein occlusion.

2.1.6.1.2 Intravitreal corticosteroids

The CRVO arm of Standard Care Versus Corticosteroid for Retinal Vein Occlusion (SCORE) study has shown that intravitreal triamcinolone acetonide (IVTA) injections of either 1 mg or 4 mg triamcinolone are effective in treating macular edema, though it is associated with the risk of raised IOP and cataract formation [21].

Randomized, Sham-Controlled Trial of Dexamethasone Intravitreal Implant in Patients with Macular Edema due to Retinal Vein Occlusion (GENEVA) study showed that 0.7 mg dexamethasone implant (Ozurdex®) can be used successfully for the treatment of macular edema. Side effects might include glaucoma and cataract [22].

2.1.6.1.3 Laser therapy

The Central Vein Occlusion Study (CVOS) states that grid photocoagulation of macula does not improve visual acuity in macular edema secondary to CRVO [23].

Delivery of panretinal photocoagulation (PRP) (**Figure 12**) is indicated at the first sign of neovascularization in CRVO [24]. But the delivery of PRP can be difficult in the eyes with NVG. So, in such scenarios anti-VEGF is used to temporarily resolve the neovascularization until PRP laser is given [25].

2.1.6.2 BRVO management

2.1.6.2.1 Intravitreal anti-VEGF therapy

Study of the Efficacy and Safety of Ranibizumab Injections in Patients with Macular Edema Secondary to Branch Retinal Vein Occlusion (BRAVO) shows the

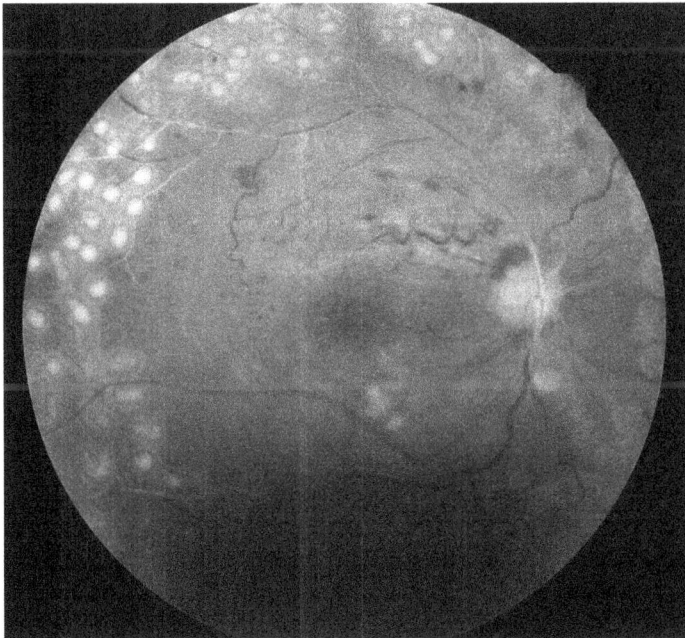

Figure 12.
Fundus photograph showing a case of CRVO treated with panretinal photocoagulation therapy.

monthly injections of 0.5 mg or 0.3 mg of ranibizumab causes improvement in macular edema and gain in visual acuity [19].

Study to Assess the Clinical Efficacy of VEGF Trap-Eye in Patients with Branch Retinal Vein Occlusion (VIBRANT) shows that aflibercept injection is useful for the treatment of CME in BRVO [26].

Comparison of Anti-VEGF Agents in the Treatment of Macular Edema from Retinal Vein Occlusion (CRAVE) shows that monthly injections of ranibizumab and bevacizumab both can be successfully used for the treatment of CME [27].

2.1.6.2.2 Intravitreal corticosteroids

The BRVO arm of the SCORE study states that macular grid laser is the benchmark for the treatment of CME when compared with IVTA injection. Grid laser is utilized with a duration of 0.1 seconds and 100 microns spot size with medium white burns [21]. IVTA was associated with elevated IOP and cataract formation [28]. Micro-pulse laser therapy is an alternative method that can be used as it causes less retinal damage, but its onset of action is slower. Though laser has been a success in macular edema secondary to BRVO, it is not effective in cases of CRVO [1].

The GENEVA study shows significant improvement of macular oedema with ozurdex implant [29].

2.1.6.2.3 Laser therapy

The Branch Vein Occlusion Study (BVOS) states that macular laser shows significant improvement in visual acuity. Scatter photocoagulation is done to treat neovascularization as it reduces the risk of vitreous hemorrhage. Laser duration of 0.1–0.2 seconds with 200–500 micron spot size of medium white burn setting is utilized [30].

Neovascularization elsewhere (NVE) or neovascularization of the disc (NVD) is considered as an indicator for sectoral photocoagulation (**Figure 7a** and **b**) in cases of BRVO [17].

2.1.7 Surgical management

Pars plana vitrectomy might prove to be beneficial in eyes with non-clearing vitreous hemorrhage in both CRVO and BRVO eyes.

2.1.8 Management of retinal vein occlusions from an emergency physician's perspective

Patients usually present to the emergency room with complaints of unilateral loss of vision, which is frequently noted on waking up in the morning. Visual acuity is usually counting fingers or worse in severe cases. RAPD elicitation is mandatory [13]. Fundus evaluation (**Figure 4a** and **b**) will show extensive dot-blot and flame-shaped hemorrhages in any one or all the quadrants depending on the level of vein occlusion. Apart from elective ophthalmic management, systemic therapy can also be initiated. Since there is no convincing evidence of systemic medical treatment in treating this condition, pilot studies have suggested the usage of oral inhibitors of platelet and erythrocyte aggregation, and hemodilution treatment to lower blood viscosity (thrombolysis) may be of some benefit. Intravenous administration of streptokinase can reduce morbidity. Unfortunately, it never gained favor because of the risk of intravitreal hemorrhage. Surgical thrombectomy is not warranted as a management option.

2.2 Ocular artery occlusions

2.2.1 Disease entity

Arterial occlusions of the eye can involve various branches. The ophthalmic artery is a branch of the internal carotid artery, which in turn gives rise to the central retinal artery and the ciliary arteries. It can either be an ophthalmic artery occlusion (OAO), a central retinal artery occlusion (CRAO), or a branch retinal artery occlusion (BRAO) (**Figure 13**) [29]. Obstruction can occur due to an embolus or a thrombus formation (Videos 3, https://www.youtube.com/watch?v=t6CwwBUl6yY and 4, https://www.youtube.com/watch?v=UnC8jo4sQgE). It can be secondary to an

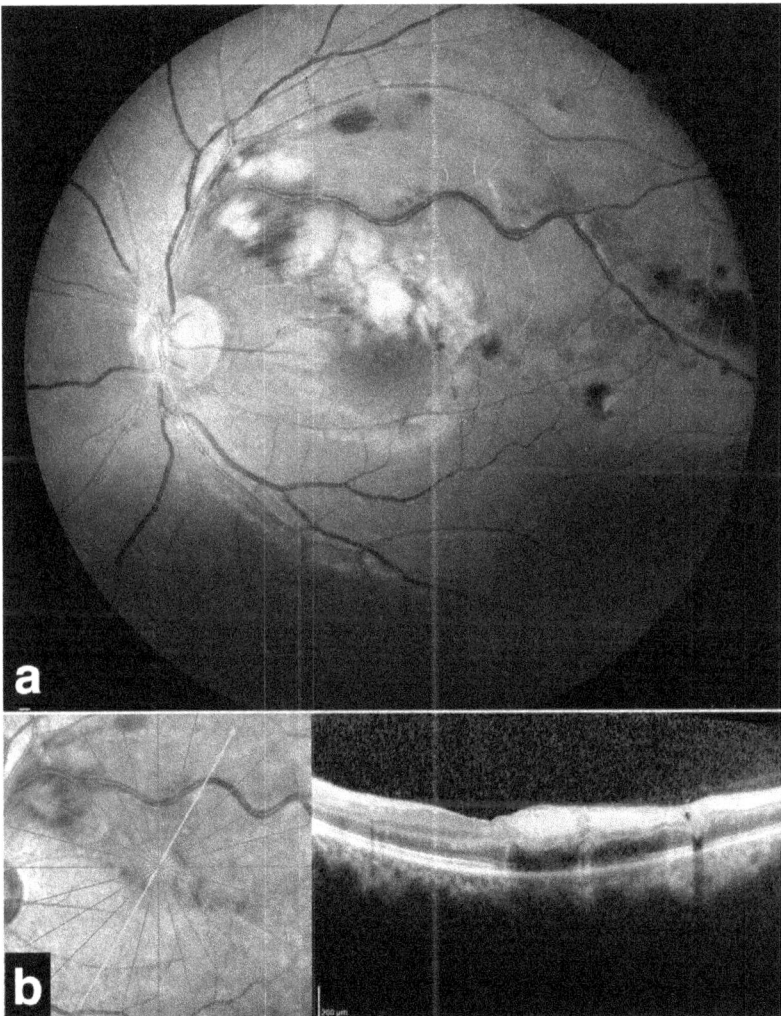

Figure 13.
(a) Fundus photograph showing BRVO with branch retinal artery occlusion (BRAO). Pale retina is seen in superotemporal aspect with tortuosity and dilatation of retinal veins, with few retinal hemorrhages and cotton-wool spots in that region. (b) OCT macula showing thickening of inner retinal layers in the superior quadrant.

inflammation of a retinal vessel wall, known as vasculitis [31, 32]. Any arterial occlusion warrants a careful systemic evaluation. Several studies have reported a strong association between retinal artery occlusions and stroke [33, 34].

Cilioretinal artery is derived from the short posterior ciliary arteries and is seen in about 15–50% of eyes. They provide blood supply to the central macula [16]. Sometimes cilioretinal artery occlusions may accompany a CRVO.

2.2.2 Central retinal artery occlusion

2.2.2.1 Etiopathogenesis

CRAO is commonly due to vascular embolic obstruction. There are several risk factors associated with retinal emboli such as shown in **Figure 14** [35, 36]. The incidence of retinal artery occlusions (RAO) increases with age and is seen more frequently in men [37, 38]. In younger patients with no atherosclerotic risk factors, conditions like vasculitis, myeloproliferative disorders, sickle cell disease, hyper-coagulable states, use of intravenous drugs or oral contraceptive pills should be explored [39]. The arteritic cause for CRAO is always due to giant cell arteritis (GCA), which has been reported in 4.5% of CRAO cases [40].

Pathophysiologies of the embolic phenomenon due to atherosclerosis is shown in **Figure 15**.

2.2.2.2 Clinical features

Patients with CRAO present with sudden, painless loss of visual acuity or a decrease in field of vision that occurs over a few seconds [41]. In 74% of the patients, visual acuity was found to be finger counting or worse with associated relative afferent pupillary defect (RAPD) [42]. If a cilioretinal artery is preserved

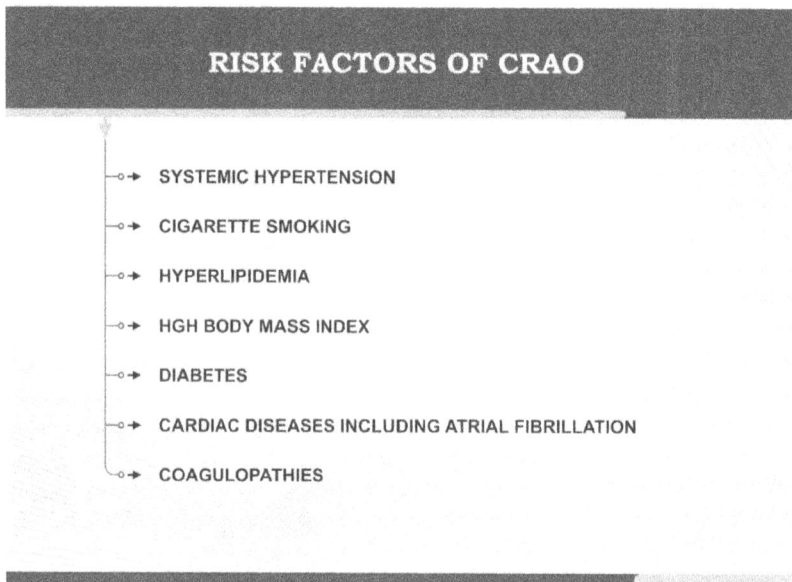

RISK FACTORS OF CRAO

- SYSTEMIC HYPERTENSION
- CIGARETTE SMOKING
- HYPERLIPIDEMIA
- HGH BODY MASS INDEX
- DIABETES
- CARDIAC DISEASES INCLUDING ATRIAL FIBRILLATION
- COAGULOPATHIES

Figure 14.
Risk factors of CRAO associated with retinal emboli.

PATHOPHYSIOLOGY OF CRAO

ATHEROSCLEROSIS

TURBULENT FLOW

DAMAGE OF THE CAROTID ENDOTHELIUM

PLAQUE DISLODGED FROM THE UNDERLYING EXPOSED CAROTID ATHEROSCLEROSIS

PLAQUE LODGE IN THE CILIO-RETINAL ARTERY

A FIBRIN-PLATELET THROMBUS MAY OR MAY NOT BE THE NIDUS FOR THE DEVELOPMENT OF A PLATELET-THROMBIN

LARGER EMBOLI MAY CAUSE A SEVERE OCCLUSION

THE ENDOTHELIUM REPAIRS THE DAMAGE PREVENTING THE PLAQUE FROM GETTING EXPOSED TO BLOOD

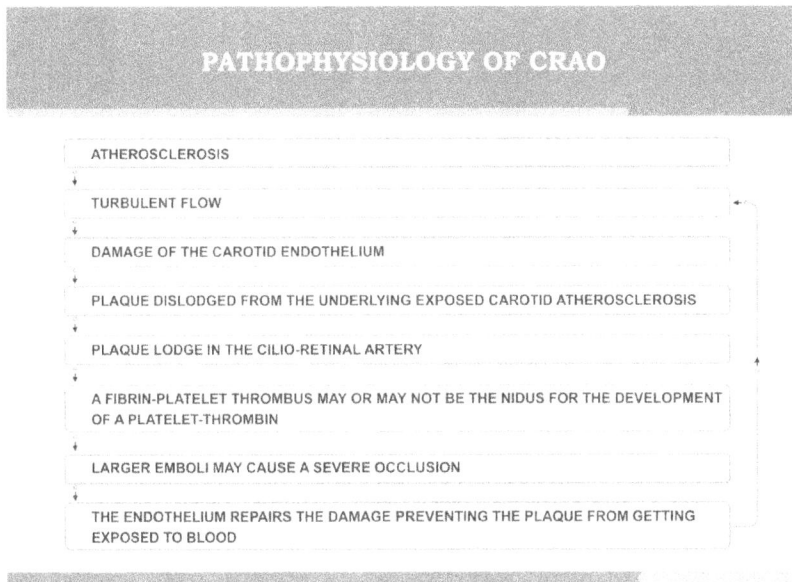

Figure 15.
Pathophysiology of an embolic phenomenon due to atherosclerosis in CRAO.

central vision will be spared [43]. Bilateral occurrence has been noted in 1 to 2% of cases [41]. An ocular examination (**Figure 16a**) can reveal the following findings: retinal opacity of the posterior pole (58%), cherry-red spot in the macula (90%), retinal arterial attenuation (32%), cattle trucking or boxcarring (19%) associated with optic disc edema (22%) and pallor (39%) [44]. An intra-arterial embolus was found in 20% of the patients, which can either be small, yellow, and refractile plaques also known as 'Hollenhorst plaque' or non-scintillating, white plaques situated in the proximal retinal vasculature due to calcific emboli, or a small pale bodies of fibrin-platelet embolus [43].

In some cases, BRAO might go unnoticed if central vision is spared.

2.2.2.3 Ocular investigations

FA shows delay in arterial filling with reduced arterial caliber, associated with masking of background choroidal fluorescence due to retinal edema. If a patent cilioretinal artery is present, it will fill during the early phase [45]. Amlaric's triangle or triangular areas of ischemia are seen in the periphery region which indicates choroidal ischemia [46].

OCT (**Figure 16b**) demonstrates an increased thickness of the inner retinal layer at the acute phase of the disease with optic disc swelling [47].

2.2.2.4 Classification

CRAO can be divided into 4 different subclasses is shown in **Figure 17**.

2.2.2.5 Systemic investigations

The battery of investigations is shown in **Figure 18**.

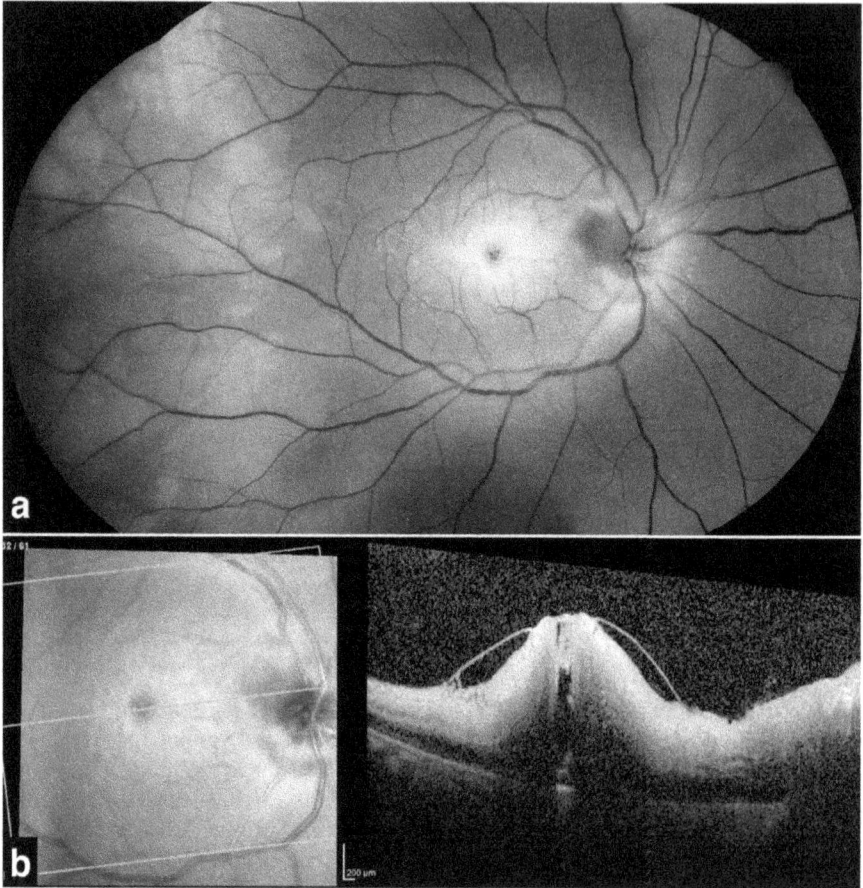

Figure 16.
Central retinal artery occlusion (CRAO). (a) Recent CRAO with the cherry-red spot in the macula with surrounding pale retina and associated disc edema. (b) OCT macula showing thickening of inner retinal layers, with thickening of the macula.

2.2.2.6 Acute management of CRAO

Significant improvement of vision is seen in only 10% of cases with spontaneous reperfusion. There are barriers involved in effective treatment because of delayed reporting of patients to the hospital and due to no consensus for guideline-based therapy [48]. The acute phase of management involves an attempt to restore the central retinal artery perfusion. It involves several non-invasive therapies and the use of intravenous or intra-arterial thrombolytics [48].

The non-invasive therapies include

- Sublingual isosorbide dinitrate, inhalation of carbogen, systemic pentoxifylline, and hyperbaric oxygen are used to dilate the retinal artery [49, 50].

- Dislodging the emboli via ocular massage [51].

- Intravenous administration of mannitol and acetazolamide along with anterior chamber paracentesis, followed by withdrawal of a small quantity of aqueous to reduce the intraocular pressure, hence increasing retinal artery perfusion [49, 52].

CENTRAL RETINAL ARTERY OCCLUSION

```
                    ┌──────────────┬──────────────────────┐
                    ↓              ↓                      ↓
          ┌──────────────────┐                  ┌──────────────────┐
          │  NON-ARTERITIC   │                  │  ARTERITIC CRAO  │
          │ PERMANENT CRAO   │                  └──────────────────┘
          └──────────────────┘
                    ↓              ↓
          ┌──────────────────┐  ┌──────────────────┐
          │  NON-ARTERITIC   │  │  NON-ARTERITIC   │
          │  TRANSIENT CRAO  │  │    CRAO WITH     │
          └──────────────────┘  │ CILIO-RETINAL    │
                                 │    SPARING       │
                                 └──────────────────┘
```

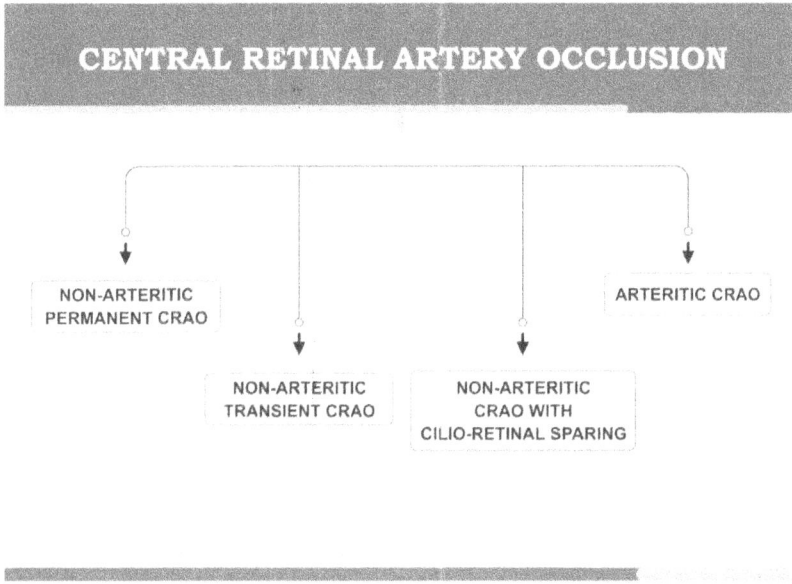

Figure 17.
Classification of CRAO.

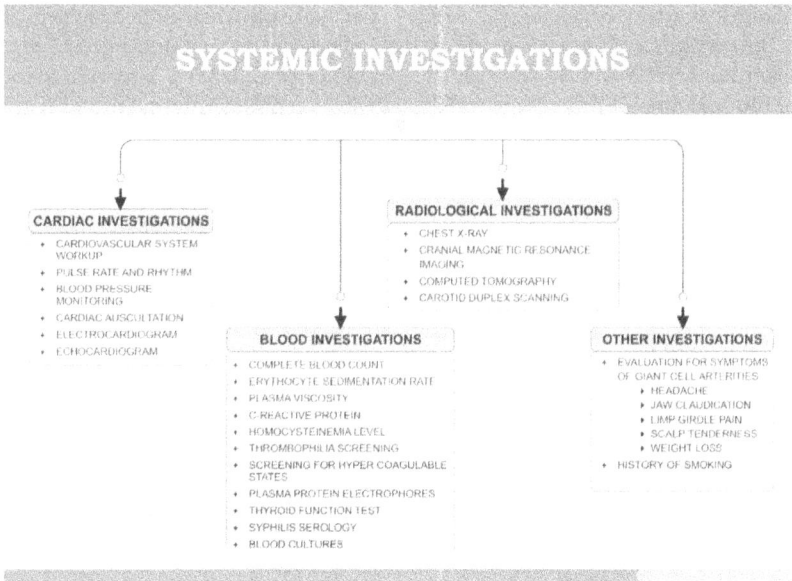

SYSTEMIC INVESTIGATIONS

CARDIAC INVESTIGATIONS
- CARDIOVASCULAR SYSTEM WORKUP
- PULSE RATE AND RHYTHM
- BLOOD PRESSURE MONITORING
- CARDIAC AUSCULTATION
- ELECTROCARDIOGRAM
- ECHOCARDIOGRAM

RADIOLOGICAL INVESTIGATIONS
- CHEST X-RAY
- CRANIAL MAGNETIC RESONANCE IMAGING
- COMPUTED TOMOGRAPHY
- CAROTID DUPLEX SCANNING

BLOOD INVESTIGATIONS
- COMPLETE BLOOD COUNT
- ERYTHOCYTE SEDIMENTATION RATE
- PLASMA VISCOSITY
- C-REACTIVE PROTEIN
- HOMOCYSTEINEMIA LEVEL
- THROMBOPHILIA SCREENING
- SCREENING FOR HYPER COAGULABLE STATES
- PLASMA PROTEIN ELECTROPHORES
- THYROID FUNCTION TEST
- SYPHILIS SEROLOGY
- BLOOD CULTURES

OTHER INVESTIGATIONS
- EVALUATION FOR SYMPTOMS OF GIANT CELL ARTERITIES
  - HEADACHE
  - JAW CLAUDICATION
  - LIMP GIRDLE PAIN
  - SCALP TENDERNESS
  - WEIGHT LOSS
- HISTORY OF SMOKING

Figure 18.
Systemic investigations done in CRAO.

Although intervention has shown improved retinal perfusion, this did not necessarily lead to improved visual acuity, and therapies do not much alter the outcome than the natural course of the disease [53]. Thrombolysis is targeted to dissolve the fibrinoplatelet occlusion in cases of non-arteritic CRAO. Several studies have shown that local intra-arterial thrombolysis has been used to re-canalize the central retinal artery, with 60–70% of the subjects responding with an improvement in visual acuity [54]. Alternatively, intravenous thrombolysis is also being administered as per standard ischemic stroke protocol. It is said to have easier access and reduced risk as compared to the intra-arterial route [55].

2.2.2.7 Sub-acute phase management of CRAO

This includes the prevention of secondary neovascular complications of the eye. Neovascularization in eyes post CRAO tends to occur between the 2nd and 16th week. Therefore, it is important to review the patient with acute CRAO at regular intervals during the first 2 weeks, followed by monthly visits for the next 4 months [56].

2.2.2.8 Long term management

The ultimate goal is to prevent other ocular ischemic events of the eye or other end organs. It is noted that 64% of patients with CRAO had at least one new vascular risk factor following the retinal occlusive event [57]. Hyperlipidemia which has been reported as the common undiagnosed vascular risk factor at the time of sentinel CRAO event should be treated chronically.

2.2.3 Cilioretinal artery occlusion

2.2.3.1 Etiopathogenesis

Cilioretinal artery occlusion (CLRAO) is the acute obstruction or blockage of blood flow within a cilioretinal artery. It typically occurs in patients aged 65 years and older but can be seen at any age. The incidence of CLRAO is approximately 1:100,000 patients [58]. It is seen unilaterally in over 99% of the cases and has no recognized hereditary pattern.
The various pathophysiological mechanisms are:

- Embolic

- Hypertensive arterial necrosis

- Inflammatory

- Hemorrhage under an atherosclerotic plaque

- Associated with concurrent central retinal vein obstruction [59]

2.2.3.2 Clinical features

2.2.3.2.1 Visual acuity

There is acute, unilateral, painless visual field loss occurring over several seconds with approximately 10% of those having a history of transient visual loss (amaurosis fugax) in the affected eye before the current episode.

2.2.3.2.2 Pupillary changes

An afferent pupillary defect may or may not be present. It entirely depends on the area of distribution of the obstruction.

2.2.3.2.3 Fundus changes

Three variants

- Cilioretinal artery obstruction (**Figure 19a**)

- Cilioretinal artery obstruction associated with central retinal vein obstruction

- Cilioretinal artery obstruction associated with acute anterior ischemic optic neuropathy [59].

2.2.3.2.4 Retinal intra-arterial emboli

Prevalence is uncertain.

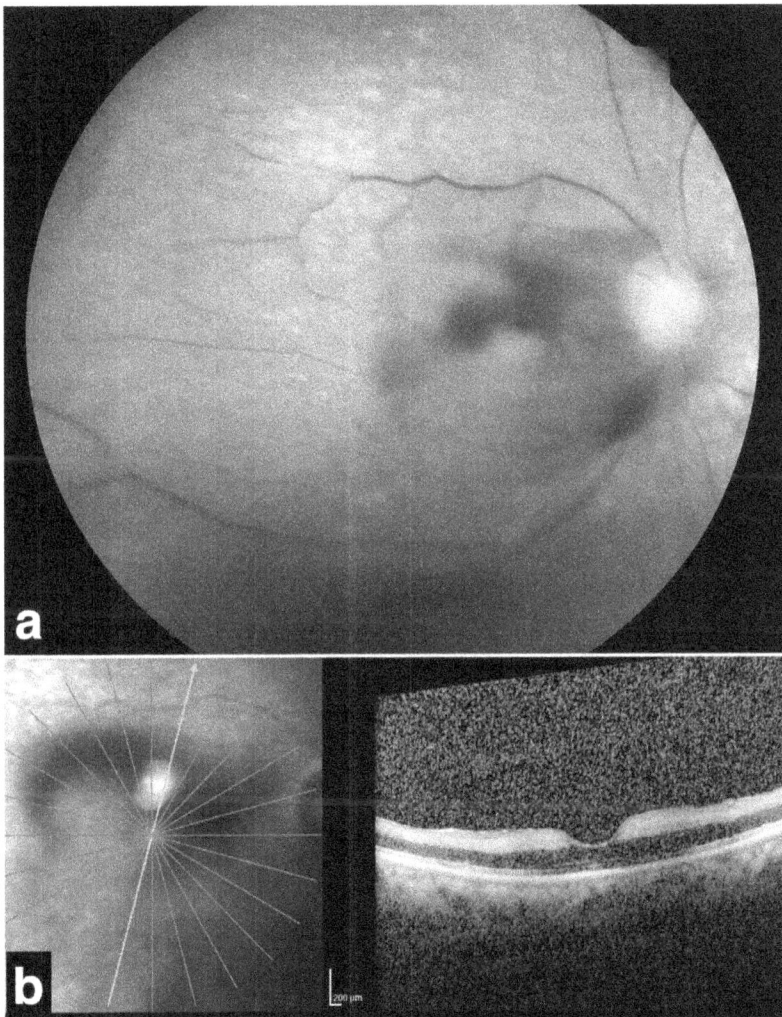

Figure 19.
(a) Fundus photograph showing cilioretinal artery obstruction with vitreous hemorrhage. (b) OCT macula image of the same showing vitreous hemorrhage and increased macular thickness with thickening of the inner retinal layers.

2.2.3.2.5 Cholesterol

It is termed as Hollenhorst plaque named after Robert Hollenhorst at the Mayo Clinic. It typically arises from the carotid arteries, which appear glistening yellow [60].

2.2.3.2.6 Differential diagnosis

- Infectious retinitis or inflammatory retinitis

- Toxoplasmosis

- Cytomegalovirus

2.2.3.3 Ocular investigations

2.2.3.3.1 Intravenous fluorescein angiography

Cilioretinal arteries normally fill with fluorescein dye during the early choroidal phase of a fluorescein angiogram. A cilioretinal artery obstruction typically shows nonperfusion of dye in the affected area throughout the retinal arteriovenous phase.

OCT macula shows increased macular thickness with thickening of the inner retinal layers (**Figure 19b**) [61].

2.2.3.4 Systemic investigations

Rule out the following:

- Causes for emboli with Carotid Doppler & Cardiac Echocardiogram

- Inflammatory causes such as Giant cell arteritis, Wegener granulomatosis, Polyarteritis Nodosa, Systemic lupus erythematous, Toxoplasmosis retinitis, Orbital Mucormycosis.

- Coagulopathies such as Lupus anticoagulant syndrome, Protein S deficiency, Protein C deficiency, Antithrombin III deficiency, Sickle cell disease, Homocystinuria.

- Miscellaneous: Fabry disease, Migraine, Lyme disease, Hypotension, Fibromuscular hyperplasia, Sydenham chorea.

2.2.3.5 Treatment

There is no consistent proven treatment to ameliorate the visual acuity. In isolated cases, even without treatment, 90% of the eyes return to 20/40 vision or better [59, 62]. With concurrent central retinal vein occlusion, 70% of eyes often return to 20/40 vision or better [63]. With anterior ischemic optic neuropathy, the vision often remains counting fingers to hand movements (HM+) despite therapy [64]. Most importantly, though uncommon, giant cell arteritis should be ruled out because, in that scenario, the fellow eye can be involved by retinal arterial obstruction within hours to days, hence hastening the need for diagnosis and treatment with high dose corticosteroids. It is essential to reduce the risk of involvement of the fellow eye [59].

2.2.4 Acute ophthalmic artery obstruction (occlusion)

2.2.4.1 Etiopathogenesis

Acute ophthalmic artery obstruction is the acute blockage of the ophthalmic artery. OAO may lead to severe ischemia of the affected globe and associated ocular structures [46]. The occlusions are usually located proximal to the branch point of the general posterior ciliary arteries and central retinal artery. Acute ophthalmic artery obstruction occurs in approximately 1:100,000 outpatient ophthalmologic visits. The mean age of onset is approximately 60 years and there is no hereditary pattern. The pathophysiological mechanism is as follows:

- Embolic

- Trauma

- Infections (Mucormycosis)

- Inflammatory (Collagen vascular disease, Giant cell arteritis)

- Dissecting Aneurysm within the ophthalmic artery

- Hemorrhage under an atherosclerotic plaque

- Vasospasm

2.2.4.2 Clinical features

2.2.4.2.1 Visual acuity

Vision loss is acute, unilateral and painless, and occurs over a period ranging from seconds to minutes. The visual acuity is no light perception in 90% of the cases.

2.2.4.2.2 Pupillary changes

An afferent pupillary defect occurs immediately.

2.2.4.2.3 Fundus changes

Superficial retinal whitening occurring in the posterior pole in acute ophthalmic artery obstruction is more pronounced than with acute retinal artery obstruction. This is because the retinal pigment epithelium may be opacified as well as with acute obstruction to the ophthalmic artery. The cherry-red spot sign may or may not be present. One-third of the patients have none, one-third of the patients have a mild cherry-red spot and another one-third of the patients have a prominent cherry-red spot.

The presence of a retinal artery embolus is variable. "Salt and Pepper" retinal pigment epithelial change can occur in the posterior pole within weeks after the acute obstruction. The pigmentary epithelial change does not occur due to central retinal artery obstruction alone.

2.2.4.2.4 Differential diagnosis

Central Retinal Artery Obstruction.

2.2.4.3 Ocular investigations

2.2.4.3.1 Intravenous fluorescein angiography

The choroid should be completely filled within 5 seconds after the injection of dye. In this condition, there will be a delay in choroidal filling. There is delayed retinal arterial and venous filling observed as well, along with late focal or diffuse staining of the retinal pigment epithelium caused by choroid ischemia.

2.2.4.3.2 Electroretinography

The a-wave is decreased or absent suggestive of outer layer retinal ischemia. The b-wave is decreased or absent suggestive of inner layer retinal ischemia.

2.2.4.4 Systemic investigations

The most common etiology is iatrogenic; occurring after retrobulbar injection. Other systemic investigations are the same as CRAO.

2.2.4.5 Treatment

Spontaneous reversal of the condition is rare. The long-term vision in most cases is usually only perception of light. There is no proven treatment yet [46]. Vigilant systemic workup is mandatory due to the lack of an effective ocular treatment. The patient should be observed closely for neovascularization for the first several months. Laser PRP should be considered if and when neovascularization develops [65].

2.2.5 Management of retinal artery occlusions from an emergency physician's perspective

The patient will present to the emergency room with acute, unilateral, painless, and severe loss of vision in the worst-case scenario. The vision loss occurs quickly within a period ranging from seconds to minutes. The visual acuity is no light perception in 90% of the cases. An afferent pupillary defect should be elicited. Fundus examination will reveal superficial retinal whitening occurring in the posterior pole in patients presenting with acute ophthalmic artery obstruction which is more pronounced than seen in patients presenting with acute retinal artery obstruction. The presence of a retinal artery embolus is variable.

Intravenous thrombolysis reduces the morbidity from acute arterial ischemic stroke pertaining to the eye, when given within 4.5 hours of the time a person was last free of symptoms [66, 67]. Intra-arterial thrombolysis is given via cannulation of the femoral artery. The introduction of a catheter is then done into the internal carotid artery, followed by the proximal ophthalmic artery at which point thrombolysis is administered. Thus, a precise dose of thrombolytic can be tailored to the individual patient in real-time. The role of surgical thrombectomy/ mechanics thrombectomy is not advocated.

2.3 Ocular ischemic syndrome

2.3.1 Disease entity

Ocular ischemic syndrome (OIS) is a result of chronic hypoperfusion, which is caused by severe ipsilateral atherosclerotic carotid stenosis, which accounts for about more than 90% of the cases. It is a rare condition [68]. It was noted that signs of ischemia were seen in both the anterior and posterior segments of the eye [69].

2.3.2 Etiopathogenesis

OIS is mostly seen in the elderly (>65 years) and men are affected twice as often as women, which is in correlation with the higher incidence of cardiovascular disease and underlying morbidity in males. Bilateral involvement is seen in 20% of the cases [70]. OIS has a five-year mortality rate of 40% mainly due to cardiac disease.

2.3.3 Clinical features

The clinical features of ocular ischemic syndrome are shown in **Figure 20** [68, 69, 71–73].

2.3.4 Investigations

FA shows prolonged arteriovenous transit time, with delayed and patchy choroidal filling, retinal vessel wall staining is present. Leakage from the disc capillaries can be present.

The most essential diagnostic tool is carotid artery imaging. Non-invasive tests like Doppler ultrasound and ocular plethysmography allow detection of stenosis in

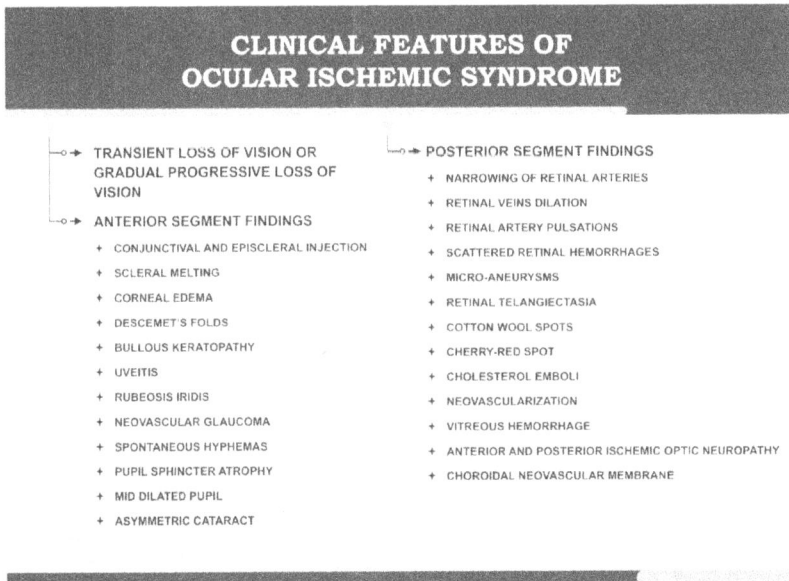

CLINICAL FEATURES OF OCULAR ISCHEMIC SYNDROME

- TRANSIENT LOSS OF VISION OR GRADUAL PROGRESSIVE LOSS OF VISION
- ANTERIOR SEGMENT FINDINGS
  - + CONJUNCTIVAL AND EPISCLERAL INJECTION
  - + SCLERAL MELTING
  - + CORNEAL EDEMA
  - + DESCEMET'S FOLDS
  - + BULLOUS KERATOPATHY
  - + UVEITIS
  - + RUBEOSIS IRIDIS
  - + NEOVASCULAR GLAUCOMA
  - + SPONTANEOUS HYPHEMAS
  - + PUPIL SPHINCTER ATROPHY
  - + MID DILATED PUPIL
  - + ASYMMETRIC CATARACT

- POSTERIOR SEGMENT FINDINGS
  - + NARROWING OF RETINAL ARTERIES
  - + RETINAL VEINS DILATION
  - + RETINAL ARTERY PULSATIONS
  - + SCATTERED RETINAL HEMORRHAGES
  - + MICRO-ANEURYSMS
  - + RETINAL TELANGIECTASIA
  - + COTTON WOOL SPOTS
  - + CHERRY-RED SPOT
  - + CHOLESTEROL EMBOLI
  - + NEOVASCULARIZATION
  - + VITREOUS HEMORRHAGE
  - + ANTERIOR AND POSTERIOR ISCHEMIC OPTIC NEUROPATHY
  - + CHOROIDAL NEOVASCULAR MEMBRANE

Figure 20.
Clinical features of ocular ischemic syndrome.

about 75% of cases. An invasive technique used is carotid arteriography, which is utilized especially before planning for surgery. In cases where Doppler ultrasound is normal, ophthalmic artery Doppler imaging should be done. Other methods such as computed tomographic angiography and magnetic resonance angiography are also used.

2.3.5 Treatment

OIS needs a multidisciplinary approach and not just an ophthalmologist. It would also require a vascular surgeon, cardiologist, neurologist, and general physician if mandated. The inflammatory component is treated with topical steroids, non-steroidal anti-inflammatory agents, and cycloplegics. In the early stages of NVG, medical management utilizing topical beta-blockers or alpha-agonists along with oral carbonic anhydrase inhibitors might be used. In cases of refractory NVG, surgical management will be required. Macular edema is either treated by IVTA or intravitreal anti-VEGF injections, but not much data regarding this treatment is available [69]. PRP is used for treatment when there is NVE, NVD and NVI in OIS.

Systemic management will include carotid endarterectomy or stenting to decrease the risk of stroke. It may even help stabilize vision by aiding in controlling NVG. In cases of total obstruction, extracranial or intracranial arterial bypass surgery will be needed [74]. Care should be taken as there is an increase in intraocular pressure (IOP) after surgery, which should be managed accordingly. Proper systemic management of cardiovascular risk factors is also mandatory.

2.3.6 Management of ocular ischemic syndrome from an emergency physician's/ intensivist's perspective

OIS needs a multidisciplinary approach. It would also require a battery of ophthalmologists, vascular surgeons, cardiologists, neurologists, and general physicians. The patient may present with complaints of transient loss of vision or gradual loss of vision with the above-mentioned fundus findings. The inflammatory component is treated with medical therapy such as topical steroids, non-steroidal anti-inflammatory agents, and cycloplegics. The surgical management includes carotid endarterectomy with no role for mechanical thrombectomy.

2.4 Cerebral venous and dural sinus thrombosis

2.4.1 Disease entity

Cerebral venous sinus thrombosis (CVST) is a clot in the venous drainage system of the brain (Video 5, https://www.youtube.com/watch?v=Y5EftYAGab0) which can result either in vision-threatening or life-threatening. Ribes MF was the first to report a case of CVST in 1825 in a 45-year-old man. The patient presented with headaches, seizures, and delirium. The autopsy confirmed cerebral venous thrombosis in the form of superior sagittal and lateral sinus thrombosis. The first postpartum autopsy confirming CVST was performed in 1828 by Abercrombie on a 25-year-old woman who died 2 weeks after an uncomplicated delivery due to CVST. Currently, the largest study exploring CVST is an Italian multi-centric study. This study involves 706 patients with CVST. The second largest study is the International Study on Cerebral Vein and Dural Sinus Thrombosis (ISCVDST) which included 624 patients with CVST [75].

2.4.2 Etiopathogenesis

CVST is an atypical stroke accounting for 0.5–1% of all strokes and affects approximately 5 per one million people annually. Cerebral Venous and Sinus Thrombosis are most commonly seen in women and children [76]. A patient presenting with CVST is more likely to be younger (less than 50 years old) when compared to typical ischemic strokes [77].

Females are at increased risk for hormone-specific risk factors such as oral contraceptives, pregnancy, and hormone replacement therapy [78]. The risk factors for CVST can be classified into genetic causes and acquired causes.

The more commonly reported etiologies of CVST are shown in **Figure 21** [79]. Virchow's triad (**Figure 22**) is the main reason behind the pathophysiology of CVST.

The thrombosis of cerebral veins occurs, most commonly in the junction between the cerebral veins and larger sinuses. The dural sinuses contain arachnoid granulations, which drain the cerebrospinal fluid (CSF) from the subarachnoid space into the systemic venous system, along with its function as venous channels. A thrombosis to the dural sinuses causes an increase in the impedance to CSF drainage resulting in increased intracranial pressure (ICP) (e.g., headache, nausea, vomiting, papilledema, and visual problems) [80].

Due to the variability in the cortical venous system, the clinical findings of a cortical vein thrombosis depend on the size of the thrombus, extent of the thrombus, location of thrombus, and nature of collateral supply. During unfavorable conditions, a CVST may lead to increased venous and capillary pressure and a breakdown in the blood–brain barrier which results in vasogenic edema, cytotoxic edema, and hemorrhage [81].

The proposed pathogenesis is explicitly shown in **Figure 23**. Commonly, both dural sinus and cortical venous thrombosis occur simultaneously, with isolation of either being very rare due to the effect of one over the other [81, 82].

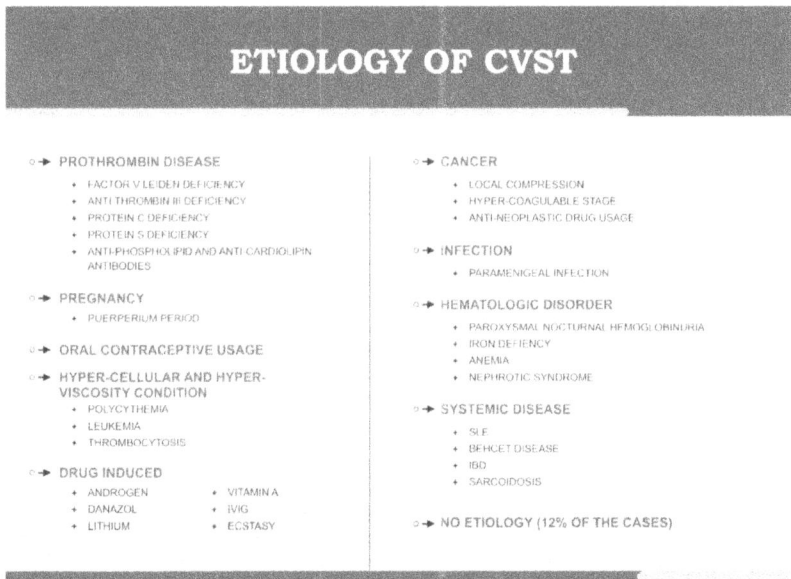

ETIOLOGY OF CVST

- PROTHROMBIN DISEASE
  - FACTOR V LEIDEN DEFICIENCY
  - ANTI THROMBIN III DEFICIENCY
  - PROTEIN C DEFICIENCY
  - PROTEIN S DEFICIENCY
  - ANTI-PHOSPHOLIPID AND ANTI CARDIOLIPIN ANTIBODIES

- PREGNANCY
  - PUERPERIUM PERIOD

- ORAL CONTRACEPTIVE USAGE

- HYPER-CELLULAR AND HYPER-VISCOSITY CONDITION
  - POLYCYTHEMIA
  - LEUKEMIA
  - THROMBOCYTOSIS

- DRUG INDUCED
  - ANDROGEN
  - DANAZOL
  - LITHIUM
  - VITAMIN A
  - IVIG
  - ECSTASY

- CANCER
  - LOCAL COMPRESSION
  - HYPER-COAGULABLE STAGE
  - ANTI-NEOPLASTIC DRUG USAGE

- INFECTION
  - PARAMENIGEAL INFECTION

- HEMATOLOGIC DISORDER
  - PAROXYSMAL NOCTURNAL HEMOGLOBINURIA
  - IRON DEFIENCY
  - ANEMIA
  - NEPHROTIC SYNDROME

- SYSTEMIC DISEASE
  - SLE
  - BEHCET DISEASE
  - IBD
  - SARCOIDOSIS

- NO ETIOLOGY (12% OF THE CASES)

Figure 21.
Etiology of cerebral venous sinus thrombosis (CVST).

VIRCHOW'S TRIAD

VENOUS STASIS

CHANGES IN
BLOOD COMPOSITION

CHANGES IN
VESSEL WALL

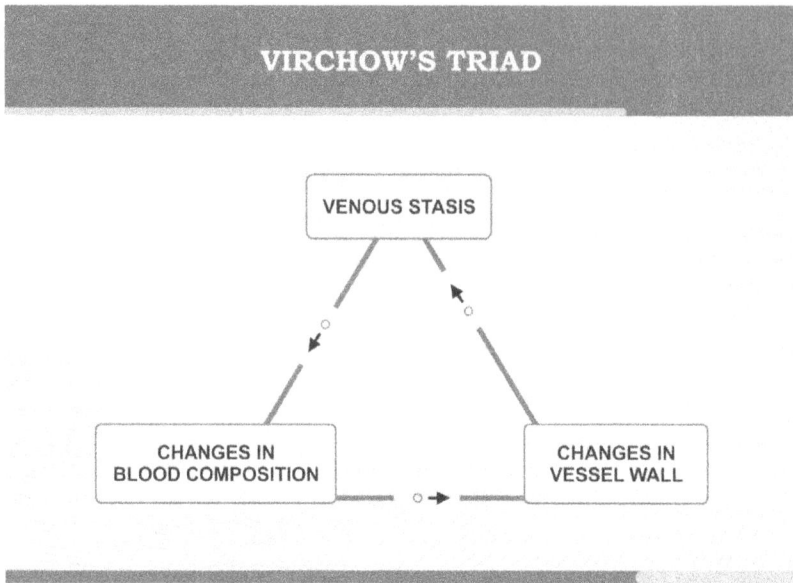

Figure 22.
Virchow's triad.

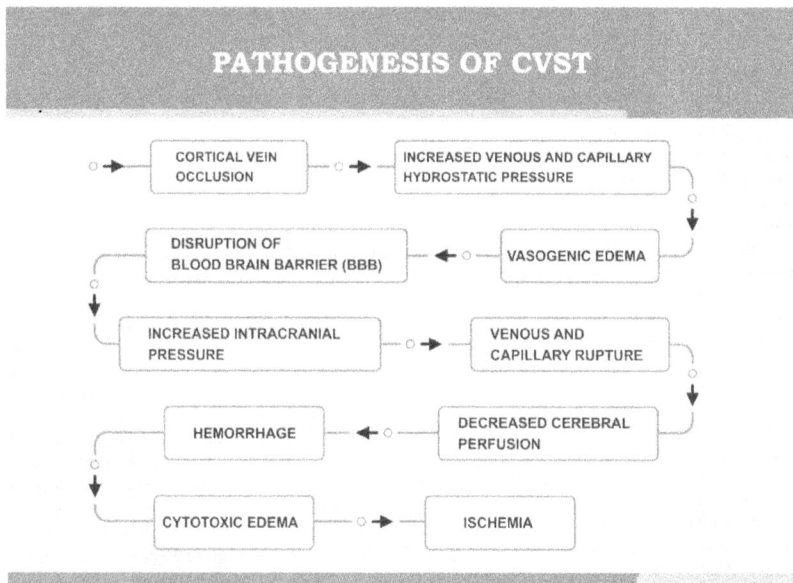

PATHOGENESIS OF CVST

CORTICAL VEIN
OCCLUSION

INCREASED VENOUS AND CAPILLARY
HYDROSTATIC PRESSURE

DISRUPTION OF
BLOOD BRAIN BARRIER (BBB)

VASOGENIC EDEMA

INCREASED INTRACRANIAL
PRESSURE

VENOUS AND
CAPILLARY RUPTURE

HEMORRHAGE

DECREASED CEREBRAL
PERFUSION

CYTOTOXIC EDEMA

ISCHEMIA

Figure 23.
Pathogenesis of CVST.

The pathophysiology causing visual impairments in CVST (**Figure 24**) is as follows:

2.4.2.1 Raised ICP without infarction

Whenever ICP increases there is a compensatory increase in CSF absorption by the arachnoid granulations. These arachnoid granulations are disrupted in dural

VISUAL IMPAIRMENTS IN CVST

→ RAISED INTRACRANIAL PRESSURE WITHOUT INFARCTION

→ VENOUS INFARCTS

→ RAISED INTRACRANIAL PRESSURE SECONDARY TO
   ARTERIOVENOUS FISTULA

→ OCCIPITAL ARTERIAL INFARCTS

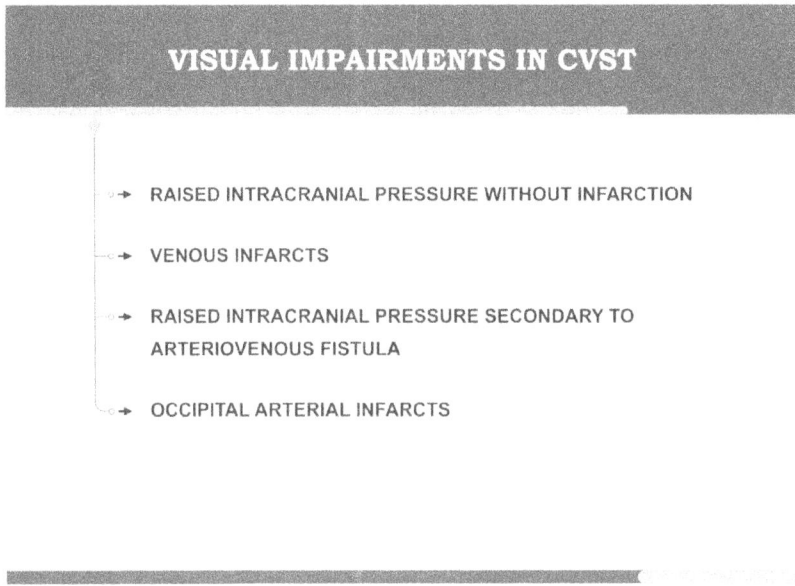

Figure 24.
Pathophysiology causing visual impairments in CVST.

sinus thrombosis. This leads to axoplasmic flow stasis with swelling of the optic nerve fiber and optic disc. The subsequent venous stasis and extracellular fluid accumulation manifest as papilledema. Patients presenting with signs and symptoms of raised ICP may be indistinguishable from idiopathic intracranial hypertension (IIH). Hence, it is mandatory that any patient with papilledema should undergo magnetic resonance imaging (MRI) of the head and a magnetic resonance venogram (MRV). Transient visual obscurations (lasting seconds at a time) or visual field defects develop due to papilledema. Diplopia may occur due to a false localizing finding of a sixth nerve palsy (**Figure 25**) due to increased ICP. Headache and pulsatile tinnitus may also occur as false localizing symptoms of increased ICP and can mimic the presentation of IIH.

2.4.2.2 Venous infarcts

Venous infarcts involve the geniculocalcarine tract especially the primary visual cortex. The involvement of occipital infarcts produces homonymous hemianopia.

2.4.2.3 Raised ICP following the development of secondary dural arteriovenous (AV) fistula

A late complication of CVST is dural AV fistula. Dural AV fistulas can cause an increase in dural sinus pressure with a subsequent decrease in CSF absorption and an increase in ICP.

2.4.2.4 Occipital arterial infarcts

Occipital arterial infarcts secondary to mass effect from the herniated large venous infarcts [83].

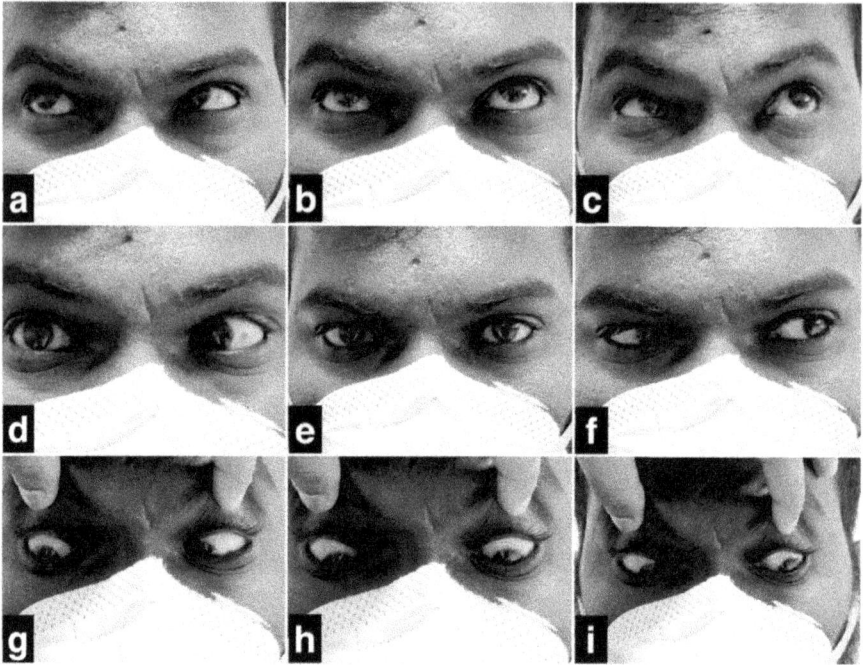

Figure 25.
(a to i) Evaluation of extraocular movements in all nine gazes showing bilateral abduction deficit (false localizing sign).

2.4.3 Clinical features

- Headache: In the ISCVDST, headache was the most common symptom (88.8%) in CVST. Headaches may be the only presenting sign, which can further complicate the diagnosis [84]. CVST in the absence of a headache is more common in older patients and men, when compared to CVST with a headache [85]. There is also a higher incidence of seizures and paresis, and a lower incidence of papilledema in CVST without a headache.

- Visual problems: Another common presenting sign/symptom in CVST according to the ISCVST is problems related to vision. Visual loss (13.2%), diplopia (13.5%), and papilledema (28.3%) were all noted. Migraine-like visual phenomena (colored photopsia, dark spots, and visual blurring associated with vertical wavy lines), have also been reported. A common finding seen in CVST is papilledema (**Figure 26**) and it is directly associated with elevated ICP. However, in eyes that have progressed to optic atrophy secondary to papilledema, the absence of papilledema cannot be used as a marker for raised ICP. Facial or craniofacial pains could be present as well.

- Seizures (39.3%): Seizures due to CVST compared to seizures due to arterial stroke (40% vs. 6%)

- Paresis (37.2%)

- Mental status changes (22%)

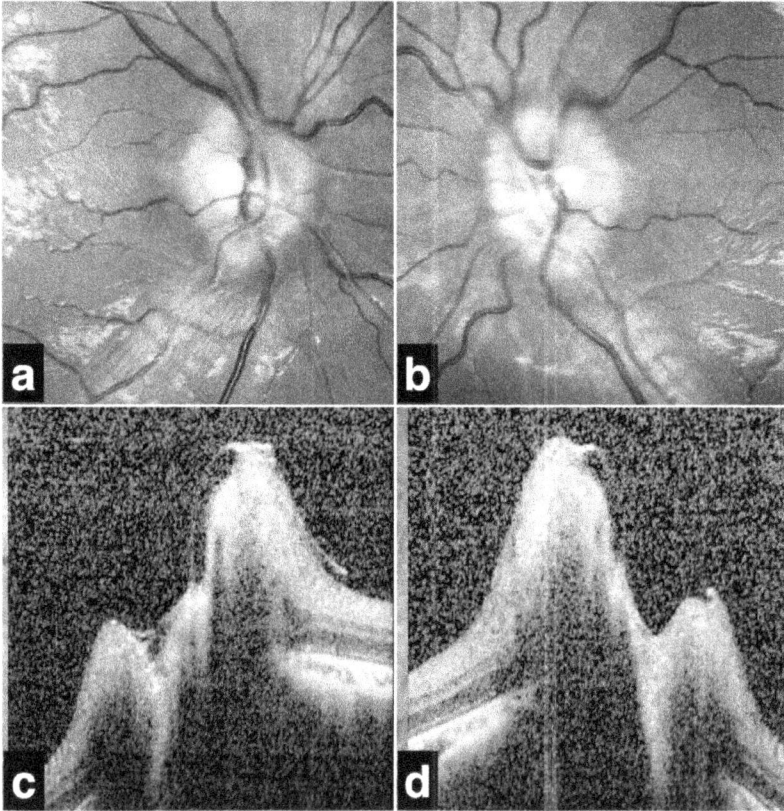

Figure 26.
(a and b) Fundus photograph showing papilledema of right (OD) and left eye (OS) respectively. (c and d) OCT optic nerve head showing disc edema of OD and OS respectively.

- Aphasia (19.1%)

- Stupor/Coma (13.9%)

- Sensory deficits (5.4%)

2.4.3.1 Clinical diagnosis

CVST has a variable clinical presentation. The diagnosis should be suspected in patients with new-onset focal neurological deficits, signs of increased ICP, seizures, or mental status changes. A thorough ocular exam comprising of dilated fundus examination, optic nerve photographs, and visual field examinations are mandatory in patients with CVST.

2.4.4 Investigations

2.4.4.1 Diagnostic imaging

The most sensitive test for identifying CVST is MRI T2 weighted imaging along with MRV. The appearance on MRI is dependent on the timeline of the thrombus. In the acute setting (days 1–5), the thrombus is typically hypointense on T2 and isointense on T1 weighted MRI. The subacute thrombosis (days 6–15) is usually strongly hyperintense on both T1 and T2 weighted images. After 3 weeks, the signal becomes irregular and either flow was restored or a persistent thrombus was seen [86].

In view of recent onset neurological deficits, a non-contrast head CT is usually the first test ordered. This test is not very specific for CVST and is abnormal in only approximately 30% of cases. In the roughly 30% of cases where CT reveals a CVST, an empty delta sign may be seen represented as a dense triangle in the posterior portion of the superior sagittal sinus (**Figure 27**). In areas where MRI/MRV are not as readily available, computed tomography venography may be added to CT to aid in the suspected diagnosis [87].

2.4.4.2 Laboratory tests

There is no laboratory study able to help rule out a CVST in the acute state [75]. However, complete blood count, chemistry panel, prothrombin time, aPTT, and a hypercoagulable state evaluation are mandatory. Testing for infectious or inflammatory states is also recommended in CVST.

2.4.4.3 Differential diagnosis

Due to the varying presentation of CVST, the differential diagnosis list (**Figure 28**) may vary according to the presenting symptom.

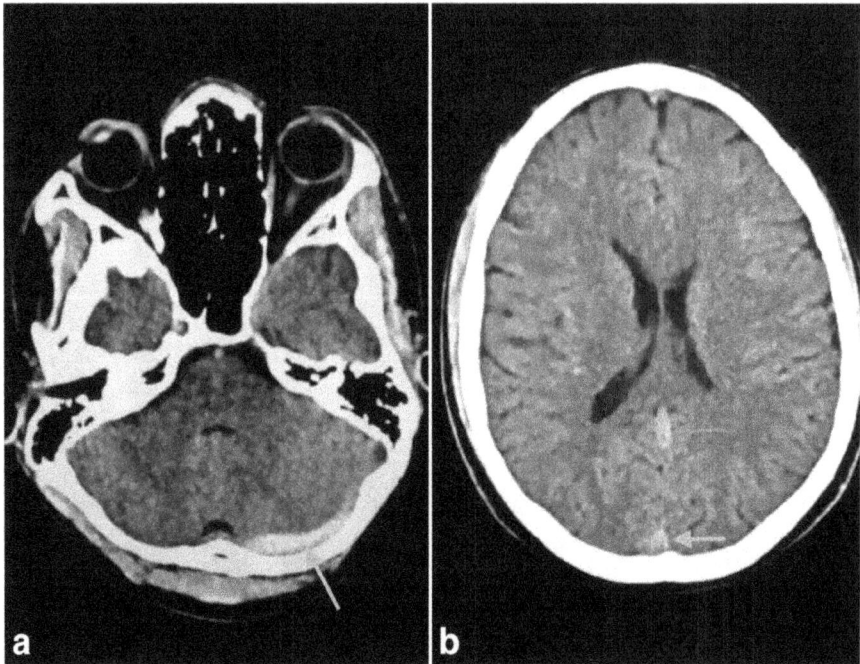

Figure 27.
Plain CT of axial section of the brain showing (a) left transverse sinus thrombosis (green arrow), (b) straight sinus thrombosis (red arrow) and superior sagittal sinus thrombosis (green arrow).

DIFFERENTIAL DIAGNOSIS OF CVST

- IDIOPATHIC INTRACRANIAL HYPERTENSION
- INTRACRANIAL TUMOUR
- BRAIN ABSCESS
- INTRACEREBRAL HEMORRHAGE
- ISCHEMIC STROKE
- MENINGOENCEPHALITIS
- AUTOIMMUNE ENCEPHALITIS
- PARANEOPLASTIC ENCEPHALITIS
- NEUROMYELITIS OPTICA

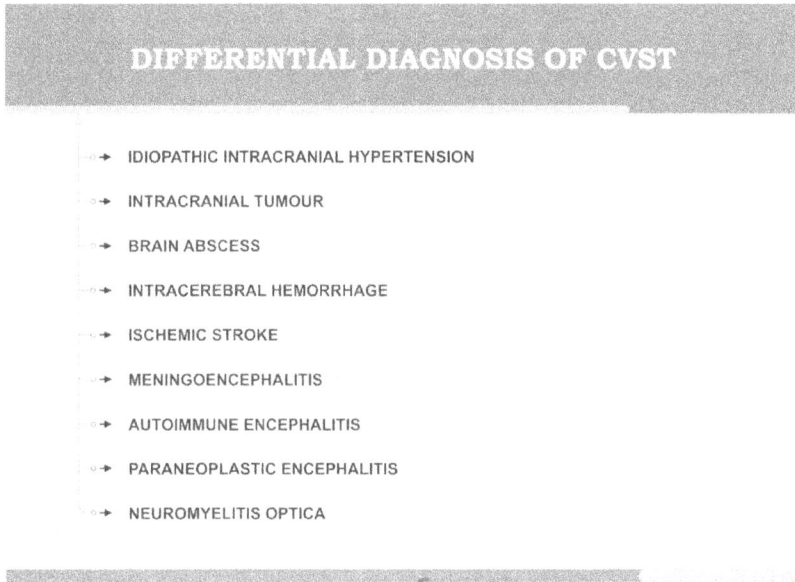

Figure 28.
Differential diagnosis of CVST.

2.4.5 Management

2.4.5.1 Medical therapy

Anticoagulation in the acute phase is preferred if there are no contraindications. Body weight adjusted subcutaneous low-molecular-weight heparin (LMWH) or dose-adjusted intravenous heparin is the drug of choice. If the patient has a concomitant intracranial hemorrhage related to the CVST, then still it is not an absolute contraindication for heparin therapy. In uncomplicated cases, LMWH is preferred over intravenous heparin due to fewer major bleeding problems. There is no evidence in the literature available for the duration of anticoagulation after the acute phase has subsided [75, 88, 89].

In cases of intracranial hypertension with secondary papilledema, progressive headache, or third or sixth nerve palsies management consists of a collection of strategies to reduce the pressure and preserve vision. The first measure is listed above; anticoagulation to reduce thrombotic occlusion of venous outflow. Other measures resemble the treatment of IIH. Serial lumbar punctures to reduce CSF volume can be considered with the caveat of needing to hold anticoagulation while it is performed. Other alternatives include treatment with acetazolamide to decrease CSF production [86]. Because blindness can be the long-term complication of elevated pressures on the optic nerve, close monitoring of visual acuity and visual fields is mandatory in patients with elevated ICP.

2.4.5.2 Surgery

Optic Nerve Sheath Fenestration (ONSF) can be planned for patients with CVST with raised ICP in situations where medical management has failed and visual function is failing. In patients where intracranial hypertension remains persistent despite adequate medical management and a lumbar drain, a CSF diversion procedure (ventriculoperitoneal or lumboperitoneal shunt) may be considered [90].

Endovascular thrombolysis and mechanical thrombectomy have not played a prominent role in the treatment of CVST but may be considered in cases of severe neurological deterioration despite the use of anticoagulation, venous infarcts causing mass effect, or intracerebral hemorrhage causing treatment-resistant intracranial hypertension [91].

2.4.5.3 Prognosis

The various prognosis of CVST is shown in **Figure 29** [92].

2.4.6 Management of CVST from an emergency physician's/intensivist's perspective

CVST has a variable clinical presentation ranging from new-onset focal neurological deficits to features suggestive of raised ICP and seizures as mentioned in the clinical features section. A thorough ocular fundus exam is mandatory in patients with CVST. It would also require a battery of vascular surgeons, neurologists, and general physicians apart from ophthalmologists.

Though the prognosis is relatively poor, coma patients in particular have been noted as a predictor of even poorer outcomes. The gold standard treatment for CVST in adults is systemic anticoagulation. The aim of anticoagulation therapy is to establish recanalization of the thrombus vessel. Emergent endovascular mechanical thrombectomy (EMT) with balloon percutaneous transmural angioplasty and catheter aspiration is indicated, in the event of failure to respond to anticoagulation or in comatose state patients. However, the role of endovascular therapy in the management of pediatric and young adult CVST is unclear [93].

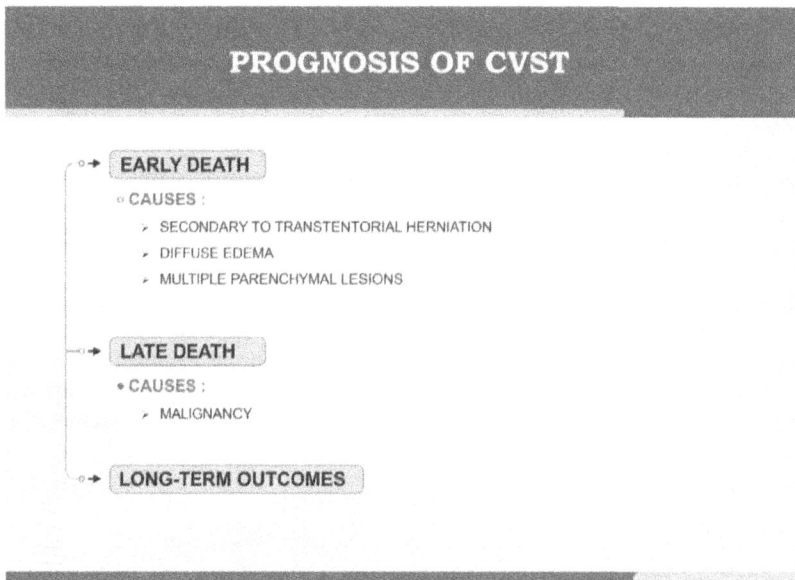

Figure 29.
Prognosis of CVST.

2.5 Cavernous sinus thrombosis

2.5.1 Disease entity

Cavernous sinus thrombosis (CST) is a condition caused by any thrombosis involving the cavernous sinus which may present as a combination of bilateral ophthalmoplegia (cranial nerves (CN) III, IV, VI), sensory trigeminal (V1-V2) loss, or autonomic dysfunction (Horner syndrome).

2.5.2 Etiopathogenesis

Patients with CST may present with ophthalmic symptoms initially to an ophthalmologist and will require urgent management considering its life-threatening prognosis. CST is typically seen as a sequela of facial infections, such as sinusitis or cellulitis. The valveless nature of the facial dural sinuses makes them vulnerable to stagnation. Poor drainage of the sinus in the setting of severe infection causes a thrombus formation. Then thrombus can cause damage to the local tissues or travel to the brain, causing stroke-like symptoms, encephalitis, or meningitis (Video 6, https://www.youtube.com/watch?v=lsSXM5SfnXE) [94].

2.5.3 Clinical features

The common clinical findings of CST are as shown in **Figure 30** [94–96].

2.5.4 Investigations

2.5.4.1 Diagnostic procedures

The diagnosis of cavernous sinus thrombosis is initially suspected on clinical grounds. However, further workup is needed to determine the underlying

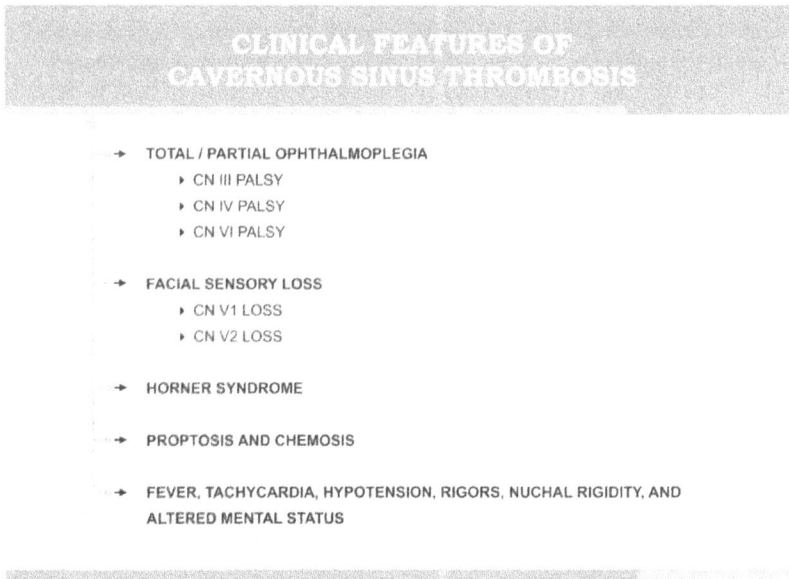

CLINICAL FEATURES OF CAVERNOUS SINUS THROMBOSIS

→ TOTAL / PARTIAL OPHTHALMOPLEGIA
  ▸ CN III PALSY
  ▸ CN IV PALSY
  ▸ CN VI PALSY

→ FACIAL SENSORY LOSS
  ▸ CN V1 LOSS
  ▸ CN V2 LOSS

→ HORNER SYNDROME

→ PROPTOSIS AND CHEMOSIS

→ FEVER, TACHYCARDIA, HYPOTENSION, RIGORS, NUCHAL RIGIDITY, AND ALTERED MENTAL STATUS

Figure 30.
Clinical features of cavernous sinus thrombosis.

pathology. Due to the wide array of potential causes, an extensive workup is warranted and called for. To confirm the diagnosis, imaging of the head and orbit, and laboratory tests play an important role.

Clinical correlation of patients' history should be done with the physical examination findings. This should be followed by appropriate diagnostic tests. Blood tests, such as complete blood count (CBC) and blood cultures are used to evaluate underlying infection. Serum studies, such as erythrocyte sedimentation rate (ESR), C-reactive protein (CRP), angiotensin-converting enzyme (ACE), and anti-neutrophil cytoplasmic antibodies (ANCA) are recommended to evaluate for an underlying inflammatory process. MRI of the brain and orbits with contrast and MRV are preferred investigations of choice to determine the presence of CST. Imaging with computed tomography (CT) of the brain and orbits or CT venography can be done as an adjunct to help adjudicate the presence of CVT [95].

2.5.5 Management

As such, treatment is not standardized but for CST recognition and timely emergency management is foremost. Intravenous antibiotics are started immediately for the treatment of any underlying infection. Though controversial, anticoagulation is recommended. Otolaryngology should be consulted to evaluate the need for surgical drainage of the primary infection [97].

2.5.6 Management of CST from an emergency physician's/intensivist's perspective

Patients with CST may initially present to an ophthalmologist but will require urgent management considering its life-threatening prognosis. Once diagnosed, this condition would warrant a battery of vascular surgeons, neurologists, and general physicians apart from ophthalmologists. CST leading to ocular hypertension and acute visual loss should be treated urgently with thrombectomy and thrombolysis of the cavernous sinuses and superior ophthalmic veins. Successful recanalization of the bilateral cavernous sinuses and superior ophthalmic veins can be achieved with transfemoral thrombectomy. Given the poor visual prognosis, if not treated urgently, recanalization with mechanical thrombectomy to immediately decrease the IOP and thus to spare the eyesight is mandatory. Anticoagulation therapy alone may not be adequate in cases of CST where vision is acutely threatened by ocular hypertension [98].

2.6 COVID-19 related/induced thrombotic ocular complications

2.6.1 Disease entity

There is a recent surge in the reporting of the various thrombotic complications related to coronavirus disease 2019 (COVID-19) in the literature, among which ophthalmology is no exception. The thromboembolic events occurring as sequela due to COVID-19 are defined as COVID-19 related/induced thrombotic ocular complication. Ophthalmologists being the first responders, have a vigilant role to play with a heightened awareness of these atypical thrombotic phenomena due to COVID-19. The incidence of a thrombotic phenomenon affecting multiple organs (with the eye being no exception) is estimated to be around 25% among patients hospitalized in the intensive care unit for COVID-19; even though anticoagulant treatment was administered prophylactically [99].

2.6.2 Etiopathogenesis

The pathophysiology of the ocular thrombotic events due to COVID-19 is linked to the complement-mediated thrombotic microangiopathy (TMA) and D-dimer levels. A potential link between mortality, D-dimer values, and the pro-thrombotic syndrome; and how it affects the end artery ocular system has been reported. Extrapulmonary thrombotic ocular manifestations are not only vision-threatening, but life-threatening too in certain instances, and are potentially treatable complications of the COVID-19.

The possible pathophysiology of the thromboembolic event is as follows: the COVID-19 virus initiates dysfunction of the endothelial cells, which in turn leads to excess thrombin generation and inhibition of fibrinolysis. This manifests with raised prothrombin levels as the end result [100]. In addition, hypoxemia is associated with an elevation of blood viscosity and activation of hypoxia-related genes that can mediate coagulation and fibrinolysis, thus favoring the fatal thrombotic events. When the plasma coagulation starts to take place, soluble fibrins are generated. This leads to the release of D-dimers which are characteristic degeneration products of cross-linked fibrin. Increased D-dimer levels trigger the activation of the coagulation cascade followed by the fibrinolytic processes.

International Federation of Clinical Chemistry Guidelines on COVID-19 strongly recommends D-dimer testing in patients with COVID-19. SARS-CoV-2 revealed a high correlation between the severity of illness and increased D-dimer levels [101, 102]. Additionally, fibrin, fibrinogen degradation products and fibrinogen are also significantly higher among patients with COVID-19.

2.6.2.1 Risk factors

2.6.2.1.1 COVID-19: the novel RNA beta-coronavirus

The novel RNA beta-coronavirus is identified as the causative pathogen for COVID-19 related/induced thrombotic ocular complications. The first infected people were exposed to live bats being sold in a wet market in Wuhan. The phylogenetic analysis revealed that bats are the potential original host of the virus.

2.6.2.2 COVID-19: the microvascular retinal circulation equation

Many different studies have shown a strong association between elevated D-dimer levels and severity of the thrombotic disease complications of COVID-19. The various thrombotic complications reported with COVID-19 are pulmonary embolism, stroke, disseminated intravascular coagulation limb infarcts, and digit infarcts [101, 102]. The involvement of the microvasculature system has created a whole new spectrum of eye diseases due to COVID-19; and the fact that retinal circulation is an end arterial system does not help. The end arterial system of the retinal vasculature is of clinical significance, because of the potential vision-threatening nature of retinal vascular diseases. Ocular manifestations have been reported to be the first sign of COVID-19 in many studies [102]. The reported ocular manifestations of COVID-19 are conjunctivitis, granulomatous anterior uveitis, choroiditis with retinal detachment, and retinal vasculitis [103].

2.6.2.3 Diabetic retinopathy-complement mediated thrombotic microangiopathy (TMA)

Zhang et al. suggested that complement-mediated thrombotic microangiopathy (TMA) is the leading factor of microvascular damage pathogenesis after COVID-19 in diabetic patients [104]. Complement system activation may be directly responsible for ocular vascular damage in accentuating diabetic retinopathy; with rare cases of atypical hemolytic uremic syndrome, leading to retinal artery, and vein occlusions [105]. High serum levels of C3 complement factor can cause an increased risk of developing diabetic retinopathy, nephropathy, and neuropathy; via endothelial dysfunction and thrombosis [106].

Immunohistochemical analysis conducted on the human eye has also revealed in favor of the 'COVID-19 induced thrombotic event' hypothesis. The ciliary body, choroid, retina, and retinal pigment epithelium (RPE) express significant levels of ACE receptors [107]. Since COVID-19 has a good affinity for vascular pericytes and expresses ACE-2, viral infection leads to complement-mediated endothelial cell dysfunction. Endothelial cell dysfunction leads to microvascular damage finally resulting in an ocular circulation infarct [108].

2.6.3 Clinical features

2.6.3.1 Retinal features

COVID-19-associated coagulopathy predisposes to a spectrum of thromboembolic events such as deep venous thrombosis, pulmonary embolism, and large-vessel ischemic strokes in patients with COVID-19. CRVO has also been described in a mechanism similar to the other thromboembolic manifestations of COVID-19. There are also cases of CRVO and CRAO being reported. The role of thrombophilic risk factors in the etiopathogenesis of retinal vein occlusions is controversial, and many authors suggest that cardiovascular risk factors for artery diseases play a more important role than coagulation disorders. The various studies reporting retinal signs and sequela post COVID-19 are shown in **Table 1**.

2.6.3.2 Optic nerve head features due to cerebral venous thrombosis

The various studies reporting optic nerve head changes and sequelae post COVID-19 are shown in **Table 2**. The optic nerve head involvement is predominantly indirect, manifesting as papilledema post cerebral venous thrombosis after COVID -19.

Study	Study sample	Inference
Marinho et al. [109]	12 adults (six males and six females, aged 25–69 years) were examined 11–33 days after the onset of COVID-19 symptoms	Hyperreflective lesion at the level of ganglion cell and inner plexiform layers at the level of papillomacular bundle
Bikdeli et al. [110]	Comprehensive Review Article	COVID-19 may predispose patients to arterial and venous thrombosis and that initial series suggest that the occurrence of venous thromboembolic disease in patients with severe COVID-19 is common

Table 1.
Retinal signs and sequelae post COVID 19 infection.

Study	Study sample	Inference
Cavalcanti et al. [111]	Three young patients, less than 41 years of age with COVID-19 had features of bilateral disc edema	COVID-19 associated cerebral venous thrombosis
Ramesh et al. [112]	A 22-year-old female patient without comorbidities presented with fever, headache, diplopia, and recurrent episodes of transient loss of vision which lasted for a few seconds in both eyes (OU) for two days. On examination, the best visual acuity was 20/20 in OU with the false localizing sign. The anterior segments were normal with bilateral disc edema, and disc hemorrhage in the right eye (OD) after the onset of COVID-19 symptoms	An unusual presentation with catastrophic cerebral venous thrombosis in previously healthy young patients infected with SARS-CoV-2 was demonstrated

Table 2.
Optic nerve signs and sequela post COVID-19 infection due to cerebral venous thrombosis.

2.6.4 Diagnostic and preventive actions

2.6.4.1 Diagnosis

The diagnosis is clinically based with laboratory investigations strengthening the association with COVID-19. The laboratory abnormalities found in COVID-19 patients include lymphopenia and elevation in lactate dehydrogenase. C-reactive protein, D-dimer, ferritin, and interleukin-6 (IL-6) have a strong correlation with disease severity and are mandatory tests in the procoagulant profile.

2.6.4.2 Role of anti-thrombotic therapy

A Chinese single-center retrospective cohort study (Tonghi hospital) of 449 consecutive patients recently concluded that severe COVID-19 patients will need prophylactic doses of heparins for improved survival (20%) especially if there is any evidence of sepsis-induced coagulopathy (SIC / DIC) [113, 114]. Severe COVID-19 was defined as either a respiratory rate $\geq$ 30/min, arterial oxygen saturation $\leq$ 93% at rest, and/or PaO2/FiO2 $\leq$ 300 mmHg. Exclusion criteria included patients with bleeding and clotting disorders, hospital stay <7 days, and lack of information on coagulation parameters and medications. Heparin was associated with lower 28-day mortality in patients with SIC/DIC.

2.6.4.3 Chest CT

To enable standardized reporting, CO-RADS were coined by the Dutch Radiological Society reporting the typical CT pattern of COVID-19 pneumonia; characterized by the consistent presence of peripheral ground-glass opacities associated with multilobar, and posterior involvement, bilateral distribution, and sub-segmental vessel enlargement [114]. Vessel enlargement described in the vicinity of ground-glass opacity areas was compatible with the thrombo-inflammatory processes [115–120]. Sub-segmental vascular enlargement (more than 3 mm diameter) in areas of lung opacity was observed in 89% of patients with confirmed COVID-19 pneumonia. All the CTs were done without contrast. Although in situ thrombosis is certainly a possibility, these findings could also represent hyperemia or increased blood flow. Anticoagulant therapy demonstrated partial or complete resolution at follow-up CT pulmonary angiography and significantly decreased mortality rates. Careful attention needs to be paid to the initial diagnosis, prevention, and treatment of the pro-thrombotic and thrombotic ophthalmic state, which can occur in a minimal but significant percentage of COVID-19 patients.

2.6.4.4 Recommendations

1. Prophylactic-dose low-molecular-weight heparin should be initiated in all patients with (suspected) COVID-19 admitted to the hospital, irrespective of risk scores especially if associated with severe vision-threatening or life-threatening ophthalmic thromboembolic conditions.

2. A baseline (non-contrast) chest CT should be considered in all patients with suspected COVID-19 with severe vision-threatening or life-threatening ophthalmic thromboembolic conditions.

3. In patients with suspected COVID-19 with severe vision-threatening or life-threatening ophthalmic thromboembolic conditions, CT pulmonary angiography should be considered, if the D-dimer level is elevated.

4. In patients with COVID-19 and severe vision-threatening or life-threatening ophthalmic thromboembolic conditions, routine serial D-dimer testing should be considered during the hospital stay for prognostic stratification.

5. COVID-induced CVST and CST should be treated urgently with thrombectomy and thrombolysis of the cavernous sinuses and superior ophthalmic veins, if they are causing ocular hypertension.

6. The role of mechanical thrombectomy is not warranted in COVID-induced retinal artery and vein occlusions.

3. Conclusions

Ocular thromboembolic complications may be the first manifestations of a life-threatening system disease or COVID-19. Ophthalmologist being the first responder needs to be vigilant and keep this possibility in mind. Heightened awareness of these atypical but life-threatening extrapulmonary treatable complications of the COVID-19 disease spectrum is encouraged and called for, especially during the time of the pandemic.

Acknowledgements

We sincerely thank Dr. Veena Shankari Padmanaban, Radiology Consultant - Anderson Diagnostics, Chennai, Tamil Nadu, India for her constant support in the interpretation of the radiological features pertaining to ocular thrombotic events. We are grateful for Mr. Pragash Michael Raj - Department of Multimedia, Mahathma Eye Hospital Private Limited, Trichy, Tamil Nadu, India for his technical support throughout the making of this chapter and its illustrations.

Conflict of interest

The authors declare no conflict of interest.

Notes/thanks/other declarations

I (Dr. Prasanna Venkatesh Ramesh) owe a deep sense of gratitude to my daughters (Pranu and Hasanna) and family (in-laws) for all their prayers, support, and encouragement. Above all, I extend my heartfelt gratitude to all the patients who consented for images which are utilized for this chapter.

Declaration of patient consent

The authors certify that they have obtained all appropriate patient consent forms. In the form, the patient(s) has/have given his/her/their consent for his/her/their images and other clinical information to be reported in the chapter. The patients understand that their names and initials will not be published and due efforts will be made to conceal their identity, but anonymity cannot be guaranteed.

Appendices and Nomenclature

INTERNATIONAL STATISTICAL CLASSIFICATION OF DISEASES AND RELATED HEALTH PROBLEMS (ICD) CODES, PERTAINING TO OCULAR THROMBOTIC PHENOMENA
  ICD-10-CM Diagnosis CodeH34 Retinal vascular occlusions
  ICD-10-CM Diagnosis Code H34.0 Transient retinal artery occlusion
      H34.00—unspecified eye
      H34.01—right eye
      H34.02—left eye
      H34.03—bilateral
  ICD-10-CM Diagnosis Code H34.1 Central retinal artery occlusion
      H34.10—unspecified eye
      H34.11—right eye
      H34.12—left eye
      H34.13—bilateral
  ICD-10-CM Diagnosis Code H34.2 other retinal artery occlusions
      H34.21 Partial retinal artery occlusion
          H34.211—right eye
          H34.212—left eye
          H34.213—bilateral
          H34.219—unspecified eye
  H34.23 Retinal artery branch occlusion
          H34.231—right eye
          H34.232—left eye
          H34.233—bilateral
          H34.239—unspecified eye
  ICD-10-CM Diagnosis Code H34.8 other retinal vascular occlusions
      H34.81 Central retinal vein occlusion
          H34.811 Central retinal vein occlusion, right eye
              H34.8110—with macular edema
              H34.8111—with retinal neovascularization
              H34.8112—stable
      H34.812 Central retinal vein occlusion, left eye
              H34.8120—with macular edema
              H34.8121—with retinal neovascularization
              H34.8122—stable

H34.813 Central retinal vein occlusion, bilateral
    H34.8130—with macular edema
    H34.8131—with retinal neovascularization
    H34.8132—stable
H34.819 Central retinal vein occlusion, unspecified eye
    H34.8190—with macular edema
    H34.8191—with retinal neovascularization
    H34.8192—stable
H34.82 Tributary (branch) retinal vein occlusion
    H34.821 Tributary (branch) retinal vein occlusion, right eye
        H34.8210—with macular edema
        H34.8211—with retinal neovascularization
        H34.8212—stable
    H34.822 Tributary (branch) retinal vein occlusion, left eye
        H34.8220—with macular edema
        H34.8221—with retinal neovascularization
        H34.8222—stable
    H34.823 Tributary (branch) retinal vein occlusion, bilateral
        H34.8230—with macular edema
        H34.8231—with retinal neovascularization
        H34.8232—stable
    H34.829 Tributary (branch) retinal vein occlusion, unspecified eye
        H34.8290—with macular edema
        H34.8291—with retinal neovascularization
        H34.8292—stable
ICD-10-CM Diagnosis Code H34.9 Unspecified retinal vascular occlusion
ICD-10-CM Diagnosis Code H35.82 Ocular Ischemic Syndrome
ICD-10-CM Diagnosis Code I67.6 Cerebral Venous Thrombosis

Nomenclature

ACE	Angiotensin-Converting Enzyme
ANA	Anti-Nuclear Antibody
AV	Arteriovenous
BBB	Blood-Brain Barrier
BP	Blood Pressure
BRAO	Branch Retinal Artery Occlusion
BRAVO	Study of the Efficacy and Safety of Ranibizumab Injections in Patients with Macular Edema Secondary to Branch Retinal Vein Occlusion
BRVO	Branch Retinal Vein Occlusion
BVOS	Branch Vein Occlusion Study
CBC	Complete Blood Count
CLRAO	Cilioretinal Artery Occlusion
COPERNICUS	Vascular Endothelial Growth Factor Trap-EyeInvestigation of Efficacy and Safety in Central Retinal Vein Occlusion Study (Conducted within North America)
COVID-19	Corona Virus Disease-2019
CRAO	Central Retinal Artery Occlusion
CRAVE	Comparison of Anti-VEGF Agents in the Treatment of Macular Edema from Retinal Vein Occlusion
C-RP	C-Reactive Protein

CRUISE	Ranibizumab for the Treatment of Macular Edema after Central Retinal Vein OcclusionEvaluation of Efficacy and Safety study
CRVO	Central Retinal Vein Occlusion
CSF	Cerebrospinal Fluid
CST	Cavernous Sinus Thrombosis
CT	Computed Tomography
CVST	Cerebral Venous Sinus Thrombosis
DIC	Disseminated Intravascular Coagulation
ECG	Electrocardiography
ESR	Erythrocyte Sedimentation Rate
FA	Fluorescein Angiography
GALILEO	Vascular Endothelial Growth Factor Trap-Eye for Macular Edema Secondary to Central Retinal Vein Occlusion Study (Conducted outside North America)
GCA	Giant Cell Arteritis
GENEVA	Global Evaluation of Implantable Dexamethasone in Retinal Vein Occlusion with Macular Edema
HM	Hand Movements
HRVO	Hemiretinal Vein Occlusion
IBD	Inflammatory Bowel Disease
ICP	Intracranial Pressure
IIH	Idiopathic Intracranial Hypertension
IOP	Intraocular Pressure
ISCVDST	International Study on Cerebral Vein and Dural Sinus Thrombosis
IVTA	Intravitreal Triamcinolone Acetonide
LMWH	Low Molecular Weight Heparin
MRI	Magnetic Resonance Imaging
MRV	Magnetic Resonance Venogram
NVD	Neovascularization of Disc
NVE	Neovascularization Elsewhere
NVG	Neovascular Glaucoma
OAO	Ophthalmic Artery
OIS	Ocular Ischemic Syndrome
ONFS	Optic Nerve Sheet Fenestration
PIRW	Peri-Venular Ischemic Retinal Whitening
PRP	Panretinal Photocoagulation
PV	Plasma Viscosity
RAO	Retinal Artery Occlusion
RAPD	Relative Afferent Pupillary Defect
RPE	Retinal Pigment Epithelium
RVO	Retinal Vein Occlusion
SCORE	The SCORE Study will compare the effectiveness and safety of standard care to intravitreal injection(s) of triamcinolone for treating macular edema (swelling of the central part of the retina) associated with central retinal vein occlusion (CRVO) and branch retinal vein occlusion (BRVO)
SIC	Sepsis Induced Coagulopathy
SLE	Systemic Lupus Erythematosus
TMA	Thrombotic Microangiopathy
VEGF	Vascular Endothelial Growth Factor
VIBRANT	Intravitreal Aflibercept for Macular Edema following Branch Retinal Vein Occlusion study

Author details

Prasanna Venkatesh Ramesh[1*], Shruthy Vaishali Ramesh[2], Prajnya Ray[3],
Aji Kunnath Devadas[3], Tensingh Joshua[4], Anugraha Balamurugan[5],
Meena Kumari Ramesh[2] and Ramesh Rajasekaran[6]

1 Department of Glaucoma and Research, Mahathma Eye Hospital Private Limited,
Trichy, Tamil Nadu, India

2 Department of Cataract and Refractive Surgery, Mahathma Eye Hospital Private
Limited, Trichy, Tamil Nadu, India

3 Department of Optometry and Visual Science, Mahathma Eye Hospital Private
Limited, Trichy, Tamil Nadu, India

4 Mahathma Centre of Moving Images, Mahathma Eye Hospital Private Limited,
Trichy, Tamil Nadu, India

5 Department of Vitreo-Retinal Surgery, Mahathma Eye Hospital Private Limited,
Trichy, Tamil Nadu, India

6 Department of Paediatric Ophthalmology and Strabismus, Mahathma Eye
Hospital Private Limited, Trichy, Tamil Nadu, India

*Address all correspondence to: email2prajann@gmail.com

IntechOpen

References

[1] Ip M, Hendrick A. Retinal Vein Occlusion Review. The Asia-Pacific Journal of Ophthalmology 2018; 7(1): 40–45.

[2] Hayreh SS. Occlusion of the central retinal vessels. Br J Ophthalmol 1965; 49(12):626–645.

[3] O'Mahoney PRA, Wong DT, Ray JG. Retinal vein occlusion and traditional risk factors for atherosclerosis. Arch Ophthalmol 2008; 126(5):692–699.

[4] Risk factors for branch retinal vein occlusion. The Eye Disease Case-control Study Group. Am J Ophthalmol 1993; 116(3):286–296.

[5] Fong AC, Schatz H, McDonald HR, Burton TC, Maberley AL, Joffe L, et al. Central retinal vein occlusion in young adults (papillophlebitis). Retina 1992; 12 (1):3–11.

[6] Hayreh SS, Zimmerman MB, Beri M, Podhajsky P. Intraocular pressure abnormalities associated with central and hemicentral retinal vein occlusion. Ophthalmology 2004; 111(1):133–141.

[7] Glacet-Bernard A, Leroux les Jardins G, Lasry S, Coscas G, Soubrane G, Souied E, et al. Obstructive sleep apnea among patients with retinal vein occlusion. Arch Ophthalmol Chic Ill 1960. 2010 Dec;128(12):1533–8.

[8] Fong AC, Schatz H. Central retinal vein occlusion in young adults. SurvOphthalmol 1993; 37(6):393–417.

[9] Lahey JM, Tunç M, Kearney J, Modlinski B, Koo H, Johnson RN, et al. Laboratory evaluation of hypercoagulable states in patients with central retinal vein occlusion who are less than 56 years of age. Ophthalmology 2002; 109(1):126–131.

[10] Morris R. Retinal vein occlusion. Kerala J Ophthalmol 2016; 28:4-13

[11] Risk factors for central retinal vein occlusion. The Eye Disease Case-Control Study Group. Arch Ophthalmol 1996; 114(5):545–554.

[12] Hayreh SS, Podhajsky PA, Zimmerman MB. Natural history of visual outcome in central retinal vein occlusion. Ophthalmology 2011; 118(1): 119-133.e1-2.

[13] Servais GE, Thompson HS, Hayreh SS. Relative afferent pupillary defect in central retinal vein occlusion. Ophthalmology 1986; 93(3):301–303.

[14] Ramesh SV, Ramesh PV. Photo quiz: Holistic integrative ophthalmology with multiplex imaging. TNOA J Ophthalmic Sci Res 2020; 58 :(33)4-5.

[15] Ramesh SV, Ramesh PV. Photo quiz answers. TNOA J Ophthalmic Sci Res 2020; 58 :(33)6.

[16] Joffe L, Goldberg RE, Magargal LE, Annesley WH. Macular branch vein occlusion. Ophthalmology 1980; 87(2): 91–98.

[17] Hayreh SS. Retinalveinocclusion. Indian Journal of Ophthalmology 1994; 42(3):109.

[18] Hayreh SS, Klugman MR, Beri M, Kimura AE, Podhajsky P. Differentiation of ischemic from non-ischemic central retinal vein occlusion during the early acute phase. Graefes Arch ClinExpOphthalmol 1990; 228(3): 201–217.

[19] Genentech, Inc. A Phase III, Multicenter, Randomized, Sham Injection-Controlled Study of the Efficacy and Safety of Ranibizumab Injection Compared With Sham in Subjects With Macular Edema Secondary to Branch Retinal Vein Occlusion [Internet]. clinicaltrials.gov; 2017 [cited 2021 Jul 28]. Available from:

https://clinicaltrials.gov/ct2/show/
NCT00486018

[20] Pielen A, Clark WL, Boyer DS, Ogura Y, Holz FG, Korobelnik J-F, et al. Integrated results from the COPERNICUS and GALILEO studies. ClinOphthalmol 2017; 11:1533–1540.

[21] Ip MS, Oden NL, Scott IU, VanVeldhuisen PC, Blodi BA, Figueroa M, et al. SCORE Study Report 3: Study Design and Baseline Characteristics. Ophthalmology 2009; 116(9):1770-1777.e1.

[22] Haller JA, Bandello F, Belfort R, Blumenkranz MS, Gillies M, Heier J, et al. Randomized, sham-controlled trial of dexamethasone intravitreal implant in patients with macular edema due to retinal vein occlusion. Ophthalmology 2010; 117(6):1134-1146.e3.

[23] Central Vein Occlusion Study (CVOS) - Full Text View - ClinicalTrials.gov [Internet]. [Cited 2021 Jul 30]; Available from: https://clinicaltrials.gov/ct2/show/ NCT00000131

[24] A randomized clinical trial of early panretinal photocoagulation for ischemic central vein occlusion. The Central Vein Occlusion Study Group N report. Ophthalmology 1995; 102(10): 1434–1444.

[25] Iliev ME, Domig D, Wolf-Schnurrbursch U, Wolf S, Sarra G-M. Intravitrealbevacizumab (Avastin) in the treatment of neovascular glaucoma. Am J Ophthalmol 2006; 142(6):1054–1056.

[26] Regeneron Pharmaceuticals. A Double-Masked, Randomized, Active-Controlled Study of the Efficacy, Safety, and Tolerability of Intravitreal Administration of VEGF Trap-Eye (IntravitrealAflibercept Injection [IAI]) in Patients with Macular Edema Secondary to Branch Retinal Vein Occlusion [Internet]. clinicaltrials.gov;

2014 [cited 2021 Jul 28]. Available from: https://clinicaltrials.gov/ct2/show/ NCT01521559

[27] Rajagopal R, Shah GK, Blinder KJ, Altaweel M, Eliott D, Wee R, et al. Bevacizumab Versus Ranibizumab in the Treatment of Macular Edema Due to Retinal Vein Occlusion: 6-Month Results of the CRAVE Study. Ophthalmic Surg Lasers Imaging Retina 2015; 46(8):844– 850.

[28] Scott IU, Ip MS, VanVeldhuisen PC, Oden NL, Blodi BA, Fisher M, et al. A randomized trial comparing the efficacy and safety of intravitreal triamcinolone with standard care to treat vision loss associated with macular Edema secondary to branch retinal vein occlusion: the Standard Care vs Corticosteroid for Retinal Vein Occlusion (SCORE) study report 6. Arch Ophthalmol 2009; 127(9):1115– 1128.

[29] Haller JA, Bandello F, Belfort R, FP 628 MS, Gillies M, Heier J, et al. Dexamethasone intravitreal implant in patients with macular edema related to branch or central retinal vein occlusion twelve-month study results. Ophthalmology 2011; 118(12):2453– 2460.

[30] Branch Vein Occlusion Study - Full Text View - ClinicalTrials.gov [Internet]. [Cited 2021 Jul 30]

[31] Ramesh SV, Ramesh PV, Ray P, Balamurugan A, Madhanagopalan V G. Photo quiz: Holistic integrative ophthalmology with multiplex imaging-part-II. TNOA J Ophthalmic Sci Res 2021;59(22)8-9.

[32] Ramesh SV, Ramesh PV, Ray P, Balamurugan A, Madhanagopalan V G. Photo answers. TNOA J Ophthalmic Sci Res 2021; 59:230.

[33] Kernan WN, Ovbiagele B, Black HR, Bravata DM, Chimowitz MI,

Ezekowitz MD, et al. Guidelines for the Prevention of Stroke in Patients With Stroke and Transient Ischemic Attack. Stroke 2014; 45(7):2160–2236.

[34] Avery MB, Magal I, Kherani A, Mitha AP. Risk of Stroke in Patients with Ocular Arterial Occlusive Disorders: A Retrospective Canadian Study. J Am Heart Assoc 2019; 8(3): e010509.

[35] Rudkin AK, Lee AW, Aldrich E, Miller NR, Chen CS. Clinical characteristics and outcome of current standard management of central retinal artery occlusion. ClinExpOphthalmol 2010; 38(5):496–501.

[36] Jauch EC, Saver JL, Adams HP, Bruno A, Connors JJB, Demaerschalk BM, et al. Guidelines for the early management of patients with acute ischemic stroke: a guideline for healthcare professionals from the American Heart Association/American Stroke Association. Stroke 2013; 44(3): 870–947.

[37] Park SJ, Choi N-K, Seo KH, Park KH, Woo SJ. Nationwide incidence of clinically diagnosed central retinal artery occlusion in Korea, 2008 to 2011. Ophthalmology 2014; 121(10):1933–1938.

[38] Park SJ, Choi N-K, Yang BR, Park KH, Lee J, Jung S-Y, et al. Risk and Risk Periods for Stroke and Acute Myocardial Infarction in Patients with Central Retinal Artery Occlusion. Ophthalmology 2015; 122(11): 2336-2343.e2.

[39] Brown GC, Magargal LE, Shields JA, Goldberg RE, Walsh PN. Retinal arterial obstruction in children and young adults. Ophthalmology 1981; 88(1):18–25.

[40] Hayreh SS, Zimmerman MB. Central retinal artery occlusion: visual outcome. Am J Ophthalmol 2005; 140 (3):376–391.

[41] Brown GC, Magargal LE. Central retinal artery obstruction and visual acuity. Ophthalmology 1982; 89(1):14–19.

[42] Varma DD, Cugati S, Lee AW, Chen CS. A review of central retinal artery occlusion: clinical presentation and management. Eye (Lond) 2013; 27 (6):688–697.

[43] Russell RW. The source of retinal emboli. Lancet 1968; 2(7572):789–792.

[44] Hayreh SS, Zimmerman MB. Fundus changes in central retinal artery occlusion. Retina 2007; 27(3):276–289.

[45] S B, Kg AE. Acute occlusion of the retinal arteries: current concepts and recent advances in diagnosis and management. Journal of accident & emergency medicine [Internet] 2000 [cited 2021 Jul 29]; 17(5).

[46] Flaxel CJ, Adelman RA, Bailey ST, Fawzi A, Lim JI, Vemulakonda GA, et al. Retinal and Ophthalmic Artery Occlusions Preferred Practice Pattern®. Ophthalmology 2020; 127(2): P259–87.

[47] Shinoda K, Yamada K, Matsumoto CS, Kimoto K, Nakatsuka K. Changes in retinal thickness are correlated with alterations of electroretinogram in eyes with central retinal artery occlusion. Graefes Arch Clin Exp Ophthalmol 2008; 246(7):949–954.

[48] Biousse V, Calvetti O, Bruce BB, Newman NJ. Thrombolysis for central retinal artery occlusion. J Neuroophthalmol 2007; 27(3):215–230.

[49] Atebara NH, Brown GC, Cater J. Efficacy of anterior chamber paracentesis and Carbogen in treating acute nonarteritic central retinal artery occlusion. Ophthalmology 1995; 102 (12):2029–2034; discussion 2034-2035.

[50] Harino S, Grunwald JE, Petrig BJ, Riva CE. Rebreathing into a bag

increases human retinal macular blood velocity. Br J Ophthalmol 1995; 79(4): 380–383.

[51] Rumelt S, Brown GC. Update on treatment of retinal arterial occlusions. CurrOpinOphthalmol 2003; 14(3): 139–141.

[52] Ffytche TJ. A rationalization of treatment of central retinal artery occlusion. Trans OphthalmolSoc U K 1974; 94(2):468–479.

[53] Margo CE, Mack WP. Therapeutic decisions involving disparate clinical outcomes: patient preference survey for treatment of central retinal artery occlusion. Ophthalmology 1996; 103(4): 691–696.

[54] Schumacher M, Schmidt D, Jurklies B, Gall C, Wanke I, Schmoor C, et al. Central retinal artery occlusion: local intra-arterial fibrinolysis versus conservative treatment, a multicenter randomized trial. Ophthalmology. 2010 Jul;117(7):1367–1375.e1.

[55] Lindsberg PJ, Mattle HP. Therapy of basilar artery occlusion: a systematic analysis comparing intra-arterial and intravenous thrombolysis. Stroke 2006; 37(3):922–928.

[56] Rudkin AK, Lee AW, Chen CS. Ocular neovascularization following central retinal artery occlusion: prevalence and timing of onset. Eur J Ophthalmol 2010; 20(6): 1042–1046.

[57] Rudkin AK, Lee AW, Chen CS. Vascular risk factors for central retinal artery occlusion. Eye (Lond) 2010; 24 (4):678–681.

[58] Hayreh SS. Acute retinal arterial occlusive disorders. ProgRetin Eye Res 2011; 30(5):359–394.

[59] Stoffelns BM, Laspas P. Cilioretinal artery occlusion.

KlinMonblAugenheilkd 2015; 232(4): 519–524.

[60] http://fyra.io. Hollenhorst Plaques [Internet]. Retina Today [cited 2021 Aug 2]; Available from: https://retina today.com/articles/2013-nov-dec/ hollenhorst-plaques

[61] Christodoulou P, Katsimpris I. Optical coherence tomography findings in a case of cilioretinal artery occlusion reversal, treated with mannitol and carbogen administration. Annals of Eye Science 2019; 4(3):13–13.

[62] Hayreh SS, Podhajsky PA, Zimmerman MB. Branch retinal artery occlusion: natural history of visual outcome. Ophthalmology 2009; 116(6): 1188-1194.e1-4.

[63] Gandhi JS, Ziahosseini K. Cilioretinal perfusion in concurrent cilioretinal and central retinal vein occlusions. Can J Ophthalmol 2008; 43 (1):121–122.

[64] Hayreh SS. THE CILIO-RETINAL ARTERIES. Br J Ophthalmol 1963; 47: 71–89.

[65] Duker JS, Brown GC. The efficacy of panretinal photocoagulation for neovascularization of the iris after central retinal artery obstruction. Ophthalmology 1989; 96(1):92–95.

[66] Tissue plasminogen activator for acute ischemic stroke. The national institute of neurological disorders and stroke rt-pa stroke study group.N Engl J Med. 1995; 333:1581–1587.

[67] Hacke W, Kaste M, Bluhmki E, Brozman M, Dávalos A, Guidetti D, et al.; ECASS Investigators. Thrombolysis with alteplase 3 to 4.5 hours after acute ischemic stroke.N Engl J Med. 2008; 359:1317–1329.

[68] Terelak-Borys B, Skonieczna K, Grabska-Liberek I. Ocular ischemic

syndrome – a systematic review. Med SciMonit 2012; 18(8):RA138–RA144.

[69] Mendrinos E, Machinis TG, Pournaras CJ. Ocular ischemic syndrome. SurvOphthalmol 2010; 55(1): 2–34.

[70] Padungkiatsagul T. Ocular Ischemic Syndrome. Journal of Thai Stroke Society 2019; 18(1):42–58.

[71] Bowling B, Kanski JJ. Kanski's clinical ophthalmology: a systematic approach. 8. ed. s.l.: Elsevier; 2016.

[72] Dugan JD, Green WR. Ophthalmologic manifestations of carotid occlusive disease. Eye 1991; 5(2): 226–238.

[73] Bogousslavsky J, Pedrazzi PL, Borruat FX, Regli F. Isolated complete orbital infarction: a common carotid artery occlusion syndrome. EurNeurol 1991; 31(2):72–76.

[74] Dzierwa K, Pieniazek P, Musialek P, Piatek J, Tekieli L, Podolec P, et al. Treatment strategies in severe symptomatic carotid and coronary artery disease. Med SciMonit 2011; 17 (8):RA191-RA197.

[75] Luo Y, Tian X, Wang X. Diagnosis and Treatment of Cerebral Venous Thrombosis: A Review. Front Aging Neurosci 2018; 10:2.

[76] Saposnik G, Barinagarrementeria F, Brown RD, Bushnell CD, Cucchiara B, Cushman M, et al. Diagnosis and Management of Cerebral Venous Thrombosis: A Statement for Healthcare Professionals From the American Heart Association/American Stroke Association. Stroke 2011; 42(4):1158–1192.

[77] Coutinho JM, Ferro JM, Canhão P, Barinagarrementeria F, Cantú C, Bousser M-G, et al. Cerebral venous and sinus thrombosis in women. Stroke 2009; 40(7):2356–2361.

[78] Bousser M-G, Ferro JM. Cerebral venous thrombosis: an update. The Lancet Neurology 2007; 6(2):162–170.

[79] Behrouzi R, Punter M. Diagnosis and management of cerebral venous thrombosis. Clin Med 2018; 18(1):75–79.

[80] Coutinho JM. Cerebral venous thrombosis. J ThrombHaemost 2015; 13Suppl 1: S238-244.

[81] Gotoh M, Ohmoto T, Kuyama H. Experimental study of venous circulatory disturbance by dural sinus occlusion. ActaNeurochir (Wien) 1993; 124(2–4):120–126.

[82] Hayreh SS. Pathogenesis of optic disc edema in raised intracranial pressure. Progress in Retinal and Eye Research 2016; 50:108–144.

[83] Aaron S, Arthur A, Prabakhar AT, Mannam P, Shyamkumar NK, Mani S, et al. Spectrum of Visual Impairment in Cerebral Venous Thrombosis: Importance of Tailoring Therapies Based on Pathophysiology. Ann Indian AcadNeurol 2017; 20(3):294–301.

[84] Cumurciuc R. Headache as the only neurological sign of cerebral venous thrombosis: a series of 17 cases. Journal of Neurology, Neurosurgery & Psychiatry 2005; 76(8):1084–1087.

[85] Coutinho JM, Stam J, Canhão P, Barinagarrementeria F, Bousser M-G, Ferro JM. Cerebral Venous Thrombosis in the Absence of Headache. Stroke 2015; 46(1):245–247.

[86] Isensee C, Reul J, Thron A. Magnetic resonance imaging of thromboseddural sinuses. Stroke 1994; 25(1):29–34.

[87] Selim M, Fink J, Linfante I, Kumar S, Schlaug G, Caplan LR. Diagnosis of Cerebral Venous Thrombosis with Echo-Planar T2*-Weighted Magnetic Resonance Imaging. Arch Neurol 2002; 59(6):1021.

[88] Einhäupl K, Stam J, Bousser M-G, De Bruijn SFTM, Ferro JM, Martinelli I, et al. EFNS guideline on the treatment of cerebral venous and sinus thrombosis in adult patients: Cerebral sinus and venous thrombosis. European Journal of Neurology 2010; 17(10):1229–1235.

[89] Ferro JM, Bousser M-G, Canhão P, Coutinho JM, Crassard I, Dentali F, et al. European Stroke Organization guideline for the diagnosis and treatment of cerebral venous thrombosis - endorsed by the European Academy of Neurology. Eur J Neurol 2017; 24(10): 1203–1213.

[90] Acheson JF. Optic nerve disorders: role of canal and nerve sheath decompression surgery. Eye 2004; 18 (11):1169–1174.

[91] Siddiqui FM, Dandapat S, Banerjee C, Zuurbier SM, Johnson M, Stam J, et al. Mechanical Thrombectomy in Cerebral Venous Thrombosis: Systematic Review of 185 Cases. Stroke 2015; 46(5):1263–1268.

[92] Canhão P, Ferro JM, Lindgren AG, Bousser M-G, Stam J, Barinagarrementeria F. Causes and Predictors of Death in Cerebral Venous Thrombosis. Stroke 2005; 36(8):1720–1725.

[93] Omoto K, Nakagawa I, Park HS, Wada T, Motoyama Y, Kichikawa K, Nakase H. Successful Emergent Endovascular Mechanical Thrombectomy for Pediatric and Young Adult Cerebral Venous Sinus Thrombosis in Coma. World Neurosurg. 2019 Feb;122:203-208.

[94] Ramesh PV, Aji K, Joshua T, Ramesh SV, Ray P, Raj PM, et al. Immersive photoreal new-age innovative gameful pedagogy for e-ophthalmology with 3D augmented reality. Indian J Ophthalmol 2022; 70: 275-280.

[95] Goyal P, Lee S, Gupta N, Kumar Y, Mangla M, Hooda K, et al. Orbital apex disorders: Imaging findings and management. Neuroradiol J 2018; 31(2): 104–125.

[96] Ebright JR, Pace MT, Niazi AF. Septic thrombosis of the cavernous sinuses. Arch Intern Med 2001; 161(22): 2671–2676.

[97] Bravo Practice Guidelines [Internet]. [Cited 2021 Jul 29]; Available from: https://www.idsociety.org/practice-guideline/practice-guidelines/

[98] Bauer J, Kansagra K, Chao KH, Feng L. Transfemoral thrombectomy in the cavernous sinus and superior ophthalmic vein. BMJ Case Rep. 2018 Feb 7;2018:bcr2017013571.

[99] Oudkerk M, Büller HR, Kuijpers D, van Es N, Oudkerk SF, McLoud T, et al. Diagnosis, Prevention, and Treatment of Thromboembolic Complications in COVID-19: Report of the National Institute for Public Health of the Netherlands. Radiology. 2020 Oct; 297(1):E216–22.

[100] Bibas M, Biava G, Antinori. A. HIV-Associated Venous Thromboembolism. Mediterr J HematolInfectDis 2011; 3(1): e2011030.

[101] Gupta N, Zhao Y-Y, Evans CE. The stimulation of thrombosis by hypoxia. Thromb Res 2019; 181:77–83.

[102] IFCC Information Guide on COVID-19 - Introduction - IFCC [Internet]. [Cited 2021 Jul 28]; Available from: https://www.ifcc.org/resources-downloads/ifcc-information-guide-on-covid-19-introduction/

[103] Seah I, Agrawal R. Can the Coronavirus Disease 2019 (COVID-19) Affect the Eyes? A Review of Coronaviruses and Ocular Implications in Humans and Animals.

OculImmunolInflamm 2020; 28(3): 391–395.

[104] Zhang Y, Xiao M, Zhang S, Xia P, Cao W, Jiang W, et al. Coagulopathy and Antiphospholipid Antibodies in Patients with Covid-19. N Engl J Med 2020; 382(17): e38.

[105] Greenwood GT. Case report of atypical hemolytic uremic syndrome with retinal arterial and venous occlusion treated with eculizumab. Int Med Case Rep J 2015; 8:235–239.

[106] Rasmussen KL, Nordestgaard BG, and Nielsen SF. Complement C3 and Risk of Diabetic Microvascular Disease: A Cohort Study of 95202 Individuals from the General Population. ClinChem 2018; 64(7):1113–1124.

[107] Sharma D, Sharma J, Singh A. Exploring the Mystery of Angiotensin-Converting Enzyme II (ACE2) in the Battle against SARS-CoV-2. Journal of the Renin-Angiotensin-Aldosterone System 2021; 2021: e9939929.

[108] Gavriilaki E, Brodsky RA. Severe COVID-19 infection and thrombotic microangiopathy: success does not come easily. British journal of hematology 2020; 189(6): e227–e230.

[109] Marinho PM, Marcos AAA, Romano AC, Nascimento H, Belfort R. Retinal findings in patients with COVID-19. Lancet 2020; 395(10237):1610.

[110] Bikdeli B, Madhavan MV, Jimenez D, Chuich T, Dreyfus I, Driggin E, et al. COVID-19 and Thrombotic or Thromboembolic Disease: Implications for Prevention, Antithrombotic Therapy, and Follow-Up: JACC State-of-the-Art Review. J Am CollCardiol 2020; 75(23):2950–2973.

[111] Cavalcanti DD, Raz E, Shapiro M, Dehkharghani S, Yaghi S, Lillemoe K, et al. Cerebral Venous Thrombosis

Associated with COVID-19. Am J Neuroradiol. 2020 Aug 1;41(8):1370–6.

[112] Ramesh SV, Ramesh PV, Ramesh MK, Padmanabhan V, Rajasekaran R. COVID-19-associated papilledema secondary to cerebral venous thrombosis in a young patient. Indian J Ophthalmol 2021; 69(3):770–772.

[113] Janssen MCH, den Heijer M, Cruysberg JRM, Wollersheim H, Bredie SJH. Retinal vein occlusion: a form of venous thrombosis or a complication of atherosclerosis? A meta-analysis of thrombophilic factors. ThrombHaemost 2005; 93(6):1021–1026.

[114] Tang N, Bai H, Chen X, Gong J, Li D, Sun Z. Anticoagulant treatment is associated with decreased mortality in severe coronavirus disease 2019 patients with coagulopathy. J ThrombHaemost 2020; 18(5):1094–1099.

[115] Caruso D, Zerunian M, Polici M, Pucciarelli F, Polidori T, Rucci C, et al. Chest CT Features of COVID-19 in Rome, Italy. Radiology 2020; 296(2): E79–E85.

[116] Frazier AA, Franks TJ, Mohammed T-LH, Ozbudak IH, Galvin JR. From the Archives of the AFIP: pulmonary veno-occlusive disease and pulmonary capillary hemangiomatosis. Radiographics 2007; 27(3):867–882.

[117] Chung MP, Yi CA, Lee HY, Han J, Lee KS. Imaging of pulmonary vasculitis. Radiology 2010; 255(2):322–341.

[118] Albarello F, Pianura E, Di Stefano F, Cristofaro M, Petrone A, Marchioni L, et al. 2019-novel Coronavirus severe adult respiratory distress syndrome in two cases in Italy: An uncommon radiological presentation. Int J Infect Dis 2020; 93: 192–197.

[119] Bai HX, Hsieh B, Xiong Z, Halsey K, Choi JW, Tran TML, et al. Performance of Radiologists in Differentiating COVID-19 from non-COVID-19 Viral Pneumonia at Chest CT. Radiology 2020;296(2): E46–E54.

[120] Ye Z, Zhang Y, Wang Y, Huang Z, Song B. Chest CT manifestations of new coronavirus disease 2019 (COVID-19): a pictorial review. EurRadiol 2020; 30(8): 4381–4389.

Chapter 7

Management of Pulmonary Thromboembolism

G. Ravi Kiran

Abstract

Pulmonary thrombo-embolism (PTE) is a major cause of cardiovascular morbidity and mortality. Incidence of PTE and its associated mortality is affected by the Prescence of associated risk factors, comorbid conditions and advancement in the treatment options. Clinical probability, D-Dimer, echocardiography and CT pulmonary angiography are used in the diagnosis. Management starts with stratification, with high-risk category being benefited from the thrombolytic therapy. Catheter directed therapy may be used in ineligible or failed cases with surgical embolectomy being used as final salvage therapy. Patients with persistent hemodynamic stability can be started on anticoagulation alone. Supportive therapy with fluid expansion and inhalational Nitric oxide may provide benefit in few. Patients with PTE should receive secondary preventive anticoagulation to prevent recurrences. High risk patients with sub-segmental PTE may benefit from anticoagulation. For early detection of long-term complications of PTE a patient cantered follow-up is needed. Chronic thrombo-embolic pulmonary hypertension (CTEPH) is a dreaded complication with pulmonary end-arterectomy being a gold standard management option in eligible patients with non-surgical therapy (balloon pulmonary angioplasty and pulmonary vasodilators) also being used in many cases.

Keywords: Pulmonary thrombo-embolism, Thrombolysis, Anti-coagulation, CTEPH, Sub-segmental PTE, Covid-19

1. Introduction

Pulmonary thrombo-embolism (PTE) is a most dangerous form of venous thrombo-embolism (VTE), and undiagnosed or untreated can be fatal. Furthermore individuals who survive PTE can develop post-PTE syndrome that is characterized by chronic thrombotic remains in pulmonary arteries, causing persistent right ventricular dysfunction, decreased quality of life and/or chronic functional limitations.

Clinical probability, assessed by validated prediction rule and age adjusted D-dimer testing is the basis for all diagnostic strategies. Computer tomographic pulmonary angiography (CTPA) is the definitive diagnostic investigation.

Acute PTE presents with varying degrees of clinical stability & thus a careful clinical assessment is needed. Patients should be evaluated in the context of various available treatment options including medical, catheter-based, and surgical interventions. Several improvements are made in therapeutic management of acute PTE in recent years.

A crisp review of the best available literature on which, multiple societal guidelines on PTE management where based, is made. Also, an evidence-based suggestions on the debatable and poorly studied PTE management topics like follow-up, sub-segmental PTE, catheter directed thrombolysis, CTEPH and covid-associated PTE were made. Areas where further need for clinical research were also highlighted.

2. Management of acute pulmonary thromboembolism

2.1 Supportive therapy

The initial approach to patients with PTE should focus on the supportive measures. It includes oxygen therapy, mechanical ventilatory support, volume expansion therapy and antibiotics (e.g., in lung infarction).

2.1.1 Volume expansion therapy

a. Expanding intra-vascular volume in patients with acute PTE is both a challenging and complicated issue.

b. In patients with moderate to severe right ventricular (RV) dysfunction; the aggressive fluid administration may lead to further increased end diastolic pressure (RVEDP) and thus leading to decreased RV coronary perfusion pressure, ultimately resulting in RV ischemia and further deterioration in RV function.

c. On the other hand, volume expansion in patients with collapsible IVC/ patients with intravascular depletion can improve cardiac output (CO). However, Identification of these 'volume responsive patients' in many times is challenging and cannot be determined with certainty.

So, in patients with no (or probably mild) RV dysfunction & when central venous pressure (CVP) is not high (< 12-15 mm Hg), then fluid therapy may be considered in hypotensive patients. However, in any case, monitoring of the RV function on a regular basis during volume expansion is recommended [1, 2].

2.1.2 Oxygen and ventilatory support

a. Patients with oxygen saturation of less than 95% in pulse oximetry must be treated with supplemental oxygen (had shown to lower RV afterload in PE). Hypoxemia can usually be controlled by oxygen inhalation.

b. In patients requiring mechanical ventilation, it is advisable to use small tidal volumes (TV) with low inspiratory pressures and low positive end expiratory pressure (PEEP) because of its adverse effect on RV function [3, 4].

2.1.3 Circulatory support

a. The ideal pharmacological agent should enhance RV function through positive inotropic effects and increase mean arterial pressure (MAP) through peripheral vasoconstriction without significantly increasing pulmonary vascular resistance (PVR).

b. The hypotensive patient with decreased cardiac output (CO) should be first started on vasopressors, and inotropes can be added later if cardiac output remains low. In contrast, inotropes can be started first in normotensive patients with evidence of decreased cardiac output, and vasopressors can be added if a hypotensive response to inotropes develops.

c. Norepinephrine can be considered a more preferable vasopressor agent for the following reasons. First, α-mediated vasoconstriction leads to increase in MAP which in turn increases right coronary perfusion pressure. Second, β1-mediated inotropic effect may improve RV function. Third, it has minimal effect on PVR.

d. Dobutamine in medium doses of up to 10 μg/kg/min can be considered as inotrope of choice. However, it should be kept in mind that, dobutamine administrated at improper high doses, increases perfusion of nonventilated regions of the lungs and may worsen respiratory insufficiency secondary to increased ventilation-perfusion (V/P) mismatch [5–7].

e. Pulmonary vasodilators like epoprostenol and inhaled nitric oxide (iNO) are shown to decrease PVR and increase CO. iNO (10–20 ppm) may be considered as a temporizing agent in patients with life-threatening PE, until therapeutic, mechanical, or spontaneous thrombolysis can be achieved and hemodynamics have improved.

Though epoprostenol causes pulmonary vasodilatation, a major concern about its use is the possible risk of worsening V/P mismatch or increasing PCWP in patients with concurrent LV dysfunction. On contrary, iNO appears to improve the V/P mismatch by increasing perfusion only to areas that are well-ventilated.

f. Based on minimal clinical data it may be suggested that if CO remains low despite vasopressors and inotropes, a pulmonary vasodilator trial with iNO may be beneficial when pulmonary hypertension is present [5–8].

Whenever possible, vasopressors and inotropic agents be used with caution, only if absolutely necessary, at the lowest possible doses.

g. Mechanical circulatory support (VA-ECMO) is sometimes may be used to provide temporary cardiopulmonary support to patients with acute cardio-pulmonary failure. In the latest ESC recommendations, ECMO was classified as "may be considered".

The Impella RP®™ (axial flow pump) and TandemHeart Protek®™ (Centrifugal pump) are RV assist devices to augment the antegrade flow; There are limited single centre reports describing the use of these devices in high-risk PTE cases [9].

To summarize the issue of supportive therapy, it can be concluded that, while used empirically based on clinical and theoretical data, there are no robust guidance emerging from the evidence-based medicine and hence needs further studies.

2.2 Medical therapy

The medical management [10–22] of acute PTE consists of anticoagulation and systemic thrombolysis.

2.2.1 Anticoagulation

a. When acute PTE is considered likely, anticoagulation should be begun while pursuing the diagnostic workup. In a hemodynamically unstable patient, it is reasonable to start anticoagulation immediately and preferably with short-acting, intravenously administered unfractionated heparin (UFH).

The rapid reversibility of IV UFH is important for these patients who may require thrombolysis or surgical embolectomy. Short-acting, intravenously administered UFH should be initiated with a bolus of 80 U/kg followed by a continuous infusion of 18 U/kg per hour.

For stable patients with PTE, low-molecular-weight heparin (LMWH) or fondaparinux are preferred to UFH due to lesser incidence of inducing major bleeding, thrombocytopenia and are associated with equal or probably superior efficacy. These agents should be continued for at least 5 days and until the INR is >2.0 for at least 24 h followed by long-term coagulation with vitamin K antagonist, VKA (the dose of warfarin should be adjusted to maintain an INR of: 2.0-3.0) or DOACs, Dabigatran and edoxaban (preferred over VKA) administered after an initial treatment of 5-10 days with LMWH.

b. As per new guidelines, haemodynamically stable patients not necessitating any thrombolytic, surgical or interventional treatment, anticoagulation can now also be started via the oral route, using one of the DOACs, apixaban or rivaroxaban (Higher doses should be used for 1 week and 3 weeks respectively).

c. Long-term anticoagulation therapy for acute PTE can be considered as 2 phasic treatments. Primary phase is for the treatment of index episode and following completion of primary treatment for the initial VTE, providers must decide whether to discontinue anticoagulant therapy or continue with long-term anticoagulation (secondary phase) with an intent to prevent VTE recurrence (secondary prevention).

d. Clinical data suggests that, all patients with PTE should receive three or more months of anticoagulant and extended oral anticoagulant reduces the risk of recurrent VTE, but the risk of bleeding partially offsets this benefit. In addition, Unprovoked PTE have a higher risk of recurrence compared to patients who had a provoked PTE (Patients with persistent risk factors are at higher risk of recurrence than those with transient risk factors).

e. Available evidence can be summarized as follows:

1. Optimal duration of anticoagulation remains uncertain and has to be considered on a case-to-case basis. In patients with provoked (identifiable risk factor) PTE, a minimum of 3 months is usually recommended, but a 6-month therapy may be considered if the patient with minor transient risk factor has low bleeding risk. Clinical data suggests against thrombophilia testing to decide the duration of anticoagulation.

2. Indefinite anticoagulation is probably appropriate for majority of the patients with unprovoked PTE (except in patients with high bleeding risk where 6 months therapy is recommended).

In certain circumstances, such as when balance between risks and benefits is uncertain, use of prognostic scores (HERDOO2, Vienna, DASH), D-dimer testing (6 month after the start of initial anticoagulation), or ultrasound assessment for residual thrombosis (after completing 6 months of anticoagulation) from an initial DVT episode may aid in reaching a final decision.

3. In cancer associated PTE, cancer is a major persistent risk factor and the need for extended anticoagulation therapy beyond 6 months is suggested for patients with an active cancer (metastatic disease) or receiving chemotherapy, provided their bleeding risk remains acceptable (low or moderate bleeding risk).

f. There is no interaction between the specific agent used and the risk of mortality, PTE. Factors such as once vs. twice-daily dosing, out-of-pocket cost, renal function, concomitant medications and the presence of cancer, may impact DOAC choice. It should be noted though there are no head-to-head trials, low quality evidence from indirect comparisons indicated that apixaban is safest DOAC.

For patients with breakthrough PTE during therapeutic VKA treatment, LMWH is preferred over DOAC therapy. For patients with concomitant stable CVD who initiate anticoagulation and were previously taking aspirin for cardiovascular risk modification, suspending aspirin over continuing it for the duration of anticoagulation therapy is recommended (not apply to patients with a recent acute coronary event or intervention).

2.2.2 Thrombolytic therapy

a. Sautter and colleagues were the among the first, who described the first successful cohort of PE patients treated with thrombolysis in 1967, demonstrating excellent clinical response with noted radiographic and hemodynamic response to therapy.

b. Thrombolytic drugs are agents that actively dissolve the thrombus & are associated with early normalization of both hemodynamic parameters and right ventricular function, but at the cost of increased risk of bleeding.

In has to be noted that even, intrinsic thrombolysis is also potent and several studies suggest that 1 week after anticoagulant therapy, the degree of vascular obstruction and right ventricular dysfunction are similar between thrombolysis-treated and anticoagulation-treated patients.

c. In clinical practice, the net benefit of thrombolysis for PTE likely exists on a continuum, highly dependent on the severity of the clinical presentation, patient's comorbidities and bleeding risk, as well as the availability of alternative therapies.

Different societal guidelines and consensus statements convey differing approaches to risk stratification, largely based on echocardiographic features and cardiac biomarkers (troponin and BNP). Systematic review data suggest that of the 17 different pulmonary embolism risk prediction scores Pulmonary Embolism Severity Index (PESI) and the simplified-PESI (sPESI) had the most robust evidence and validation for clinical risk assessment of patients with PTE.

d. Data from randomized trials and systematic literature reviews suggest that:

1. Presence of hemodynamic instability (defined as systolic blood pressure < 90 mm Hg for 15 minutes or more) is the most important determinant of short-term mortality and represents a high-risk cohort. So, these patients should receive immediate systemic thrombolytic therapy (TT) though the evidence on the mortality benefit is of only low quality.

2. In hemodynamically stable PTE patients presenting with both RV dysfunction and elevation of myocardial injury markers (troponins and BNP) are classified as intermediate-high–risk PE. Early thrombolysis in this group prevents hemodynamic decompensation which was offset by the higher bleeding events and the net effect on mortality is controversial.

In light of this evidence, full-dose systemic TT is routinely recommended for intermediate-high risk PTE and should be only be reserved as rescue therapy for those presenting with clinical deterioration after initial anticoagulation.

Because the bleeding risk associated with TT is dose dependent, lower doses of thrombolytic drugs may provide a more favorable safety profile with comparable efficacy. In fact, in a systematic review, low-dose tPA was associated with lower risk of major bleeding than full-dose tPA, with no difference in recurrent PTE.

Thus, in low bleeding risk patients (ex. young, < 65 kg) with intermediate high-risk PTE, low-dose systemic thrombolysis (with tPA) at presentation may result in the net favorable outcomes & should be considered (PEITHO-III [NCT04430569] is an ongoing placebo-controlled RCT evaluating the mortality benefit of this approach).

3. TT is effective if applied within the first 48 hours of symptom onset. Its efficacy decreases significantly after 7 days, but it may be beneficial up to 14 days from symptom onset.

4. Data on the use of systemic TT in patients with PTE-related cardiopulmonary arrest, patients at high risk for decompensation due to concomitant cardio-pulmonary disease and free thrombus in the right ventricle or atrium are limited, and probably a case-based approach is recommended.

e. Three different thrombolytics have FDA approval for PTE: urokinase as a 4400-IU/kg intravenous (IV) bolus, followed by a 4400-IU/kg/h infusion over 12 to 24 hours; streptokinase via a 250,000-IU IV loading dose over 30 minutes, followed by 100,000 IU/h over 12 to 24 hours.

Alteplase is the most commonly administered thrombolytic agent. Although the FDA-approved dose of 100 mg of alteplase over 2 hours is most commonly used, European and Canadian guidance supports the option of alteplase 0.6 mg/kg administered over 15 minutes.

Though not approved many studies had shown the efficiency of reteplase (2 bolus doses of 10 U each, 30 min apart) and tenecteplase (single bolus dose of 0.5 mg/Kg) in treating pulmonary embolism.

Only few comparison trials of available thrombolytic agents have been conducted. Available data suggest a clinical superiority of tenecteplase over streptokinase, alteplase over urokinase and streptokinase. Further studies are needed to truly identify the choice of thrombolytic agent and regimen in PTE.

2.3 Catheter directed therapies

a. Catheter-directed therapy provides an alternative reperfusion approach that allows localized drug delivery and can be combined with mechanical thrombus removal that may result in better clinical outcomes.

Catheter-based therapies include MT, mechanical thrombectomy (thrombus fragmentation, aspiration, rheolytic thrombectomy), Pharmacologic catheter directed thrombolysis (CDT, via thrombolytic infusion catheter or ultrasound-facilitated CDT), or a combination of both.

b. Different techniques of MT include [23, 24]

1. Thrombus maceration (Using a pigtail catheter or guidewire). However, distal embolization may be an inadvertent risk.

2. Rheolytic thrombectomy using AngioJet®™ device uses rapid-speed saline that facilitate thrombus fragmentation. The catheter can also be used to deliver low-dose thrombolytic agent into the thrombus to aid clot removal.

3. Aspiration thrombectomy using FlowTriever®™ device is the first MT procedure approved by FDA. The Indigo Thrombectomy CAT 8 system®™ and AngioVac®™ catheter are other systems used for this purpose.

c. Endovascular thrombolysis is done by placement of a multi-hole catheter within the pulmonary artery (PA) and infusing a thrombolytic agent (most commonly used is tPA, at a rate of 0.5–1 mg/h per catheter when 2 catheters are used, or 0.5–2 mg/h when only 1 catheter is used) for 12-24 hours.

1. To improve the efficacy and speed of clot clearance, fibrinolysis can be combined with low-intensity ultrasound waves (EkoSonic Endovascular System®™) in an approach called ultrasound-assisted thrombolysis [25]. However, there is no clear evidence demonstrating the benefit of ultrasound-enhanced thrombolysis over standard CDT. On the contrary, the procedure times are significantly longer than for standard CDT [26–28].

2. The major advantage of CDT over systemic thrombolysis is lower bleeding risk [25]. In fact, in a meta-analysis of outcomes of CDT, the rates of major bleeding were significantly lower were compared to systemic thrombolysis in patients with high- and intermediate-risk patients. However, current evidence supporting the use of CDT in acute PTE is limited to a small RCTs or single-arm studies focusing on short-term surrogate outcomes rather than long-term clinical outcomes.

3. Due to lack of strong RCT evidence regarding the short- and long-term clinical benefits, based on the critical review of meta-analytic and clinical studies it may be suggested that [26–32]:

In patients with high-risk PTE, CDT is recommended when systemic thrombolysis is contraindicated or has failed or as alternative in high bleeding risk patients (e.g., coagulopathy).

Though in Intermediate-risk PTE, CDT is associated with lower mortality with equivalent rates of major bleeding compared to systemic anti-coagulation alone, quality of evidence is not robust. CDT may thus be reserved for these patients who develop signs of hemodynamic instability despite adequate anticoagulation as an alternative to systemic thrombolysis in case-to-case basis.

Additional studies with larger sample sizes are required to elucidate the optimal use of CDT in sub-massive PTE.

2.4 Surgical pulmonary embolectomy

a. Surgical pulmonary embolectomy was associated poor outcome as it is performed only as a lifesaving therapy. Systematic review data suggest that in-hospital mortality rate in patients undergoing the procedure was around 25% with a better value of about 15% from recent studies.

b. It is useful to treat patients with massive PTE when other methods are contraindicated or fail and when the patient presents a relatively low surgical risk. It may be also used when there is a large proximal or intracardiac thrombi with a risk of paradoxical embolism via a patent foramen ovale, in expert surgical centres [33, 34].

2.5 Follow-up

a. Care for patients with acute PTE after discharge includes attention aimed at prevention of major bleeding, identification of underlying disease, and monitoring for long-term complications. Timing of follow-up is based on the patient's characteristics and the ideal time for the initial visit must be individualized, and generally ranges from 2 weeks to 3 months.

b. There are no guidelines for post-PTE imaging due to lack of clinical trials. But available small-scale data suggests that:

1. Though the gold standard technique for assessing the pulmonary arterial hypertension (PAH) is right heart catheterization (RHC). TTE (transthoracic echocardiography) should always be performed at discharge to evaluate PAH. TTE at follow-up (at 3 months) should be considered only for those patients with RV–RA gradient >45 mmHg or in the presence of both dyspnoea and a RV–RA gradient ranging between 32 and 45 mmHg at discharge.

2. Lung perfusion scan must be performed 3 months after the acute event in those patients with persisting symptoms and/or in the presence of right ventricular dysfunction or pulmonary artery hypertension.

3. Computed tomography of pulmonary vasculature and pulmonary vascular MRI are not useful to define therapeutic strategies during the follow-up and are thus not recommended.

c. Thrombophilia testing in its current form does not significantly impact clinical management or improve outcomes for most VTE patients. Data strongly suggest against testing in provoked PTE, where as in unprovoked PTE there is only limited data to suggest the benefit of testing and is usually not recommended except in those patients with a positive familiar history of VTE or recurrent thrombosis or suspecting APLA syndrome.

Though ESC guidelines recommend against the use of DOAC in APLA syndrome, recent systematic review suggests that rate of VTE recurrence and bleeding events were both low and comparable in patients with various thrombophilia receiving VKA or DOAC suggesting that DOAC are appropriate treatment option even in this population.

d. Extensive screening for occult cancer in every patient with unprovoked VTE is not recommended, however guidelines suggest a limited screening strategy though clinically significant benefit of this approach is unknown.

"Limited screening strategy" includes medical history, physical examination and laboratory analyses with blood cell count, renal and liver function parameters and calcium levels as well as a simple chest x-ray. In addition, according to national recommendations, specific screening based on sex and age (colon, breast, cervical and prostate) should be performed [35–41].

However, some patients with high-risk features (RIETE score of >3 may benefit from extensive cancer screening with CT imaging. Prospective validation of this approach is still being tested (SOME RIETE, NCT03937583 & MVTEP2-SOME2, NCT04304651 trails).

3. Prophylaxis

3.1 Medical prophylaxis

a. Many meta-analysis that includes both observational and intervention studies suggest a beneficial effect of statin use for prevention (primary and secondary) of VTE. In intervention studies, therapy with rosuvastatin significantly reduced VTE (including PTE) compared with other statins.

But scientific committees feel it is still too early to make any guideline recommendations based on the current evidence [42, 43].

b. Guidelines suggest that hospitalized patients who have an active malignancy should receive pharmacologic thromboprophylaxis (combined regimen of pharmacologic and mechanical prophylaxis may improve efficacy) in the absence of contraindications. However, routine thromboprophylaxis generally not be offered to patients admitted for minor procedures or chemotherapy infusion [44].

c. Risk of VTE is high in patients undergoing major orthopedic surgeries like a knee or hip surgeries. At least 10-14 days, preferably 35 days from the day of surgery, pharmacological thromboprophylaxis is recommended in the absence of risk factors for bleeding.

For assessing VTE risk is patients undergoing non-orthopedic surgery, modified Caprini risk assessment score is used. Based on this assessment score, patients with moderate to high-risk should receive pharmacological prophylaxis (+/− mechanical methods).

d. Although data comparing pharmacologic prophylaxis to placebo is of low quality, major clinical practice guidelines still recommend pharmacologic VTE prophylaxis for almost all acute medical critically illness.

Commonly used pharmacological agents for prophylaxis are: UFH, LMWH & Fondaparinux (later two are usually preferred over UFH) [45].
Duration of DVT prophylaxis is typically until the patients can ambulate or discharge from the hospital. In patients undergoing abdominal or pelvic surgery for cancer and with a low risk of bleeding, pharmacological prophylaxis is extended to a total duration of 4 weeks [45].

3.2 IVC filters

a. Because majority of emboli to pulmonary circulation arise from deep veins of legs, use of IVC filter (retrievable or non-retrievable) was emerged as a therapy for preventing PTE.

b. In clinical practice, clinicians use them in diverse VTE population, like patients with poor compliance to anticoagulant use, limited cardio-pulmonary reserve, large free-floating proximal DVT and also in patients with high risk of VTE prophylactically [46].

In-fact, meta-analytic data suggest that the IVC filters were associated with reduction of recurrent PE but causes increased risk of DVT, and albeit no significant effect on PTE-related or overall mortality [47, 48].

c. In should be noted that majority of the evidence for the use of IVC filters in people with VTE was of very low quality, which is majorly insufficient to make any strong recommendations.

Expert consensus based on all the available evidence recommend not to offer IVC filters to people with DVT or PTE unless it is part of a clinical trial or was covered by their other recommendations for people in whom anticoagulation is contraindicated or who have PTE taking appropriate anticoagulation treatment.
Systematic review [49] suggests that IVC filters with cylindrical or umbrella elements have highest reported risk of IVC thrombosis compared to conical filters, clinical relevance of this is yet to be studied.

4. Hot topics in PTE

4.1 Isolated sub-segmental pulmonary embolism

ISSPE is defined as a contrast defect in a sub-segmental artery, that is, the 1st arterial branch of any segmental artery independent of artery diameter.

a. With the advent of improved technology in CTPA, there is a better visualization of peripheral vessels, thereby increasing the detection rate if subsegmental pulmonary embolism (SSPE) and it accounts for 15% of all PE diagnosis recently.

b. Data suggest that ISSPE is not usually associated with adverse clinical outcomes and mortality, leading to an ongoing debate on the need for anticoagulation in these patients. In a systematic review, comparison of the pooled clinical data from uncontrolled outcome studies shows no increase in VTE recurrence for patients who were not anticoagulated compared to patients who received anticoagulation.

c. However, some patients may be at higher risk of recurrent events. A clinical expert panel favors anticoagulation treatment in case of prior VTE, APLAS - antiphospholipid syndrome, active cancer and proximal DVT [50–54].

4.2 Covid associated PTE

a. A major concern in patients with severe COVID-19 pneumonia is concomitant prothrombotic state known as COVID-19-associated coagulopathy (CAC) and its pathophysiology centres around the bidirectional model of thrombosis and inflammation (thrombo-inflammation). Systematic review data suggest that:

1. The frequency of PTE in patients with COVID-19 is highest in the ICU (25-50%), followed by general wards (15-25%). PTE in COVID-19 is more commonly located in peripheral than in central pulmonary arteries, which suggests local thrombosis to play a major role. Increasing age & body mass index was associated with an increasing prevalence of PTE.

2. Patients with PTE had significantly higher D-dimer levels and a D-dimer assessment may help to select patients with COVID-19 for CTPA, using D-dimer cut-off levels of at least 1000 µg/L (cut-off levels which have been used to identify patients with PE varied between 1000 and 4800 µg/L in different studies). The odds of mortality are significantly higher among patients who developed PTE compared to those who did not.

b. Data from low-quality studies, show that in adult hospitalized patients AC, anticoagulation is associated with improved pulmonary oxygenation, decreased coagulopathy markers and decreased mortality.

Though Anticoagulation dosing varied throughout the studies and may be classified as standard VTE prophylaxis, intermediate dosing, or full dose AC. Limited data also suggests that therapeutic doses might be associated with better survival compared to prophylactic doses.

However, at present, no randomized data is available to support one approach over another. Based on the available clinical evidence it may be suggested that

1. Routine thrombo-prophylaxis with SC heparin (UFH or LMWH) may be recommended in all adult hospitalized (in particular ICU) patients with standard VTE prophylactic dose provided there are no contraindications. LMWH can be preferred over UFH (to limit exposure) and DOACs (to limit drug interactions).

2. Considering a 50% increase in the dose in obese patients (>120 kg or BMI > 40 kg/m^2) and using therapeutic dose in patients on mechanically ventilation or proven VTE event (present or past).

Though little data suggested D-dimer driven escalated thrombo-prophylaxis - i.e. Using therapeutic anticoagulation in patients with very high D-Dimer levels (ex. > 3.0 µg/ml) or significantly rising D-dimer levels (ex. > 0.5 µg/ml per day) even after prophylactic dosing; may improve clinical outcomes, large scale studies are needed and presently daily monitoring of d-dimer for the purpose of guiding anticoagulant therapy is not recommended (but, worsening clinical status in conjunction with rising D-dimer, may necessitate the escalation of anticoagulation therapy). In should be noted that a French guidance document recommends full-therapeutic dose anticoagulation for patient with increase in fibrinogen to >8 g/l or D-dimer of >3.0 µg/ml.

3. Due to the absence of the clinical studies, use of antiplatelet agents for VTE prevention should not be used based on data from non-covid-19 patients. Addition of mechanical thrombo-prophylaxis to pharmacological agents may be considered in critically ill patients.

4. Physical activity and ambulation should be recommended to all discharged patients when appropriate. Extended VTE prophylaxis should be considered in patients with documented VTE event. In others though elevated d-dimer levels (greater than twice the upper limit of normal), in addition to comorbidities such as cancer and immobility, may help to risk stratify there is no clinical guidance in whom VTE prophylaxis be given and may be only considered on case-to-case basis (up to 6 weeks); because, cumulative incidence of a VTE episode in the post-acute COVID-19 setting is <5% at 30-45 days follow-up.

COVID-19 patients who are at low bleeding risk (VTE-Bleed score < 2 or Orbit score < 3) and were admitted to the ICU, intubated, sedated, and possibly paralyzed for multiple days may get benefited from out-of-hospital prophylaxis.

c. So, at this point of time, full role of therapeutic-dose anticoagulation must be further elucidated in the settings of larger RCT. Furthermore, whether heparin-based anticoagulants are superior to DOAC or VKA in terms of clinical outcome in patients with COVID-19 requires further study. Agent of choice (DOACs vs. enoxaprin), indications and duration of post-covid thromboprophylaxis need to be further evaluated. Role of antiplatelet agents such as aspirin as an alternative (or in conjunction with anticoagulation agents) for thromboprophylaxis in COVID-19 has not yet been defined.

d. In critically ill COVID-19 hemodynamically stable patients (systolic blood pressure, SBP >90 mmHg) with documented PE, parenteral AC might be preferred to oral anticoagulant therapy (LMWH may be preferred over UFH except in patients with severe renal dysfunction and/or with high bleeding risk) due to frequent association of drug interactions, GI and kidney dysfunction. Challenges for thrombolytic therapy in hemodynamically unstable (SBP <90 mmHg for >15 minutes) covid-19 patients:

1. Coagulopathy associated with covid changes from supressed-fibrinolytic (elevated D-dimer, normal fibrinogen) to enhanced-fibrinolytic type (elevated D-dimer, decreased fibrinogen) during the disease progression and thrombolytic therapy (TT) may be dangerous in the later type.

2. Due to critically ill nature of disease, cause for hemodynamic instability cannot ascertained to PTE with certainty in all.

3. Associated comorbid condition (GI and kidney dysfunction) may increase attendant bleeding risk with TT.

Though there is a scare data on the efficiency of inhalation therapy with fibrino-lytic substances in PTE in general, they should be used only in clinical trial settings and in all other situations TT (systemic thrombolysis using a peripheral vein over CDT) should be considered in high-risk PTE patients when other causes of instability are reasonably excluded [55–65].

5. Management of CTEPH

CTEPH is major cause of chronic pulmonary hypertension leading to right heart failure and death. Lung ventilation/perfusion scintigraphy is the screening test of choice; a normal scan rules out CTEPH. In the case of an abnormal perfusion scan, a high-quality pulmonary angiogram is necessary to confirm and define the pulmonary vascular involvement and prior to making a treatment decision. Its management principles are [66–73]:

a. After the diagnosis of CTEPH was made patients should receive diuresis for volume overload and supplemental oxygen for hypoxemia if indicated.

b. Pulmonary end-arterectomy (PEA) is considered as a gold-standard treatment in eligible patients. CTEPH operability has to be assessed by experienced CTEPH multidisciplinary teams.

   Systematic review data suggest that only 60% of CTEPH cases are operable and in 25% of operated patients, pulmonary hypertension persists; for whom non-surgical alternative therapies (BPA and Pulmonary vasodilator therapy) must be considered, because they were shown to improve pulmonary hemodynamics and 6-minute walk distance (6MWD). However, their impact on mortality is yet to be proven.

c. Pulmonary vasodilators: Endothelin receptor antagonists (ERA: Oral Bosentan & macitentan), Soluble guanylate cyclase stimulators (Riociguat), Prostanoids (Epoprostonil IV, trepostinil SC), PDE5i (sildenafil) are used. Only Riociguat (Soluble guanylate cyclase stimulator) remains the only approved medical therapy for CTEPH patients deemed inoperable or with persistent PH after PEA [34].

d. Balloon pulmonary angioplasty (BPA) is an interventional angiographic procedure in which stenotic segmental and subsegmental pulmonary arteries are dilated using a standard balloon angioplasty technique.

   Though, preliminary encouraging data suggests that BPA might have higher survival rate with fewer complication rate compared with PEA [74], at this point of time CTEPH still remains the standard therapy for operable CTEPH cases and guidelines state that BPA may be considered for patients who are technically inoperable or who carry an unfavorable risk/benefit ratio for PEA.

e. Anticoagulation: Lifelong anticoagulation is routinely recommended and used in CTEPH to prevent recurrent venous thromboembolism. The ideal choice of anticoagulation agent has not been established.

Multi-centre data suggested that the use of DOAC therapy resulted in a higher incidence of PTE recurrence compared with VKA without any survival difference.

Although, there are an emerging positive data regarding the efficacy of DOAC therapy in this setting, standard practice is to use VKA (target INR of 2-3).

6. Important relevant latest guidelines

See references [75–82].

7. Conclusion

a. Management of acute PTE starts with risk stratification based on (s)PESI scoring and the patients with hemodynamic instability should receive systemic thrombolysis (ST). Patients with intermediate-high risk PTE may be thrombolysed if they deteriorate after initial anticoagulation or upfront low dose ST may be considered particularly if the patient has no high bleeding risk.

However, choice of thrombolytic agent and evidence-based indications to stop ST in indicated patients is largely unknown.

b. Both catheter-based therapies (CBT) and surgical pulmonary embolectomy (SPE) are well accepted second line therapies in patients who have failed ST. However, comparative effectiveness of these approaches is difficult to study with systematic review data suggesting significantly higher absolute mortality with SPE compared to CBT.

Based on the available evidence catheter directed thrombolysis (CDT) may be considered as 2nd line therapy in appropriate patients, if ST fails. Use of CDT in sub-massive PE need further evidence to define its appropriate role.

c. DOACs should be preferred to VKA for the long-term management of PTE with available evidence suggesting similar efficiency of all 4 DOACs and relatively lower bleeding risk with apixaban. There is no routine role of thrombophilia testing in PTE and in almost all do not alter our choice of preferring DOACs over VKA.

d. Management of sub-segmental PE is ongoing hot-debate with limited RCT data. Expert opinion is not to anticoagulate the patient until the patient has high risk features like proximal lower limb DVT.

Further studies are in need of the hour to identify the significance of subsegmental PE and appropriate candidates for systemic anticoagulation.

e. Appropriate follow-up of PTE patients is clinically very important for early recognition of CTEPH, which is managed with surgical end-arterectomy is eligible patients and in others, non-surgical therapies like balloon pulmonary angioplasty or pulmonary vasodilator therapy with available evidence suggesting a clinical superiority of former therapy.

f. Statins may be considered for secondary prophylaxis in PTE patients. Primary prophylaxis with heparin (UFH or LMWH) should be considered in appropriate patients with acute medical illness, active cancer and high-risk surgeries.

Use of IVC filters is based on low quality evidence and at present may be inserted in only a subset of PE patients (ex. contra-indication for anticoagulation) as secondary prophylaxis.

g. Covid associated PTE is related to thrombo-inflammation and routine prophylaxis with standard dose of LMWH is recommended in all hospitalized patients and role of therapeutic dose of LWWH as prophylaxis in yet to be properly defined. Extended VTE prophylaxis in patients with no documented in-hospital VTE episode should be considered on case-to-case basis.

Ongoing clinical trials will shed more light on the role of aspirin for VTE prophylaxis, dose and duration of AC for VTE prophylaxis in hospitalized and non-hospitalized patients.

Conflict of interest

None to declare.

Author details

G. Ravi Kiran
Department of Cardiology, Government General Hospital,
Kurnool, Andhra Pradesh, India

*Address all correspondence to: drrxrk@gmail.com

IntechOpen

References

[1] Mercat A, Diehl JL, Meyer G, Teboul JL, Sors H. Hemodynamic effects of fluid loading in acute massive pulmonary embolism. Crit Care Med. 1999 Mar;27(3):540-544.

[2] Schouver ED, Chiche O, Bouvier P, Doyen D, Cerboni P, Moceri P, Ferrari E. Diuretics versus volume expansion in acute submassive pulmonary embolism. Arch Cardiovasc Dis. 2017 Nov;110(11): 616-625.

[3] Kline JA, Hernandez-Nino J, Newgard CD, Cowles DN, Jackson RE, Courtney DM. Use of pulse oximetry to predict in-hospital complications in normotensive patients with pulmonary embolism. Am J Med. 2003;115:203-208.

[4] Lyhne MD, Hansen JV, Dragsbæk SJ, Mortensen CS, Nielsen-Kudsk JE, Andersen A. Oxygen Therapy Lowers Right Ventricular Afterload in Experimental Acute Pulmonary Embolism. Crit Care Med. 2021 Apr 19.

[5] Bělohlávek J, Dytrych V, Linhart A. Pulmonary embolism, part II: Management. Exp Clin Cardiol. 2013;18(2):139-147.

[6] Barco S, Konstantinides SV. Pulmonary Embolism: Contemporary Medical Management and Future Perspectives. Ann Vasc Dis. 2018;11(3):265-276. doi:10.3400/avd. ra.18-00054.

[7] Martinez Licha CR, McCurdy CM, Maldonado SM, Lee LS. Current Management of Acute Pulmonary Embolism. Ann Thorac Cardiovasc Surg. 2020;26(2):65-71. doi:10.5761/atcs. ra.19-00158.

[8] Bhat T, Neuman A, Tantary M, Bhat H, Glass D, Mannino W, Akhtar M, Bhat A, Teli S, Lafferty J. Inhaled nitric oxide in acute pulmonary embolism: a systematic review. Rev Cardiovasc Med. 2015;16(1):1-8.

[9] Elder M, Blank N, Shemesh A, et al. Mechanical Circulatory Support for High-Risk Pulmonary Embolism. Interv Cardiol Clin. 2018 Jan;7(1):119-128. doi: 10.1016/j.iccl.2017.09.002.

[10] Yamamoto T. Management of patients with high-risk pulmonary embolism: a narrative review. J Intensive Care. 2018;6:16. Published 2018 Mar 2. doi:10.1186/s40560-018-0286-8.

[11] Barco S, Konstantinides SV. Pulmonary Embolism: Contemporary Medical Management and Future Perspectives. Ann Vasc Dis. 2018;11(3):265-276. doi:10.3400/avd. ra.18-00054.

[12] Martinez Licha CR, McCurdy CM, Maldonado SM, Lee LS. Current Management of Acute Pulmonary Embolism. Ann Thorac Cardiovasc Surg. 2020;26(2):65-71. doi:10.5761/atcs. ra.19-00158.

[13] Rivera-Lebron B, McDaniel M, Ahrar K, PERT Consortium et al. Diagnosis, treatment and follow up of acute pulmonary embolism: consensus practice from the PERT Consortium. Clin Appl Thromb Hemost. 2019;25:1076029619853037. doi: 10.1177/1076029619853037.

[14] Zuo Z, Yue J, Dong BR, et al. Thrombolytic therapy for pulmonary embolism. Cochrane Database Syst Rev. 2021 Apr 15;4(4):CD004437. doi: 10.1002/14651858.CD004437.pub6.

[15] Chatterjee S, Chakraborty A, Weinberg I, et al. Thrombolysis for pulmonary embolism and risk of all-cause mortality, major bleeding, and intracranial hemorrhage: a meta-analysis. JAMA. 2014 Jun

18;311(23):2414-2421. doi: 10.1001/jama.2014.5990.

[16] Riera-Mestre A, Becattini C, et al. Thrombolysis in hemodynamically stable patients with acute pulmonary embolism: a meta-analysis. Thromb Res. 2014 Dec;134(6):1265-1271. doi: 10.1016/j.thromres.2014.10.004.

[17] Konstantinides SV, Vicaut E, Danays T, et al. Impact of Thrombolytic Therapy on the Long-Term Outcome of Intermediate-Risk Pulmonary Embolism. J Am Coll Cardiol. 2017 Mar 28;69(12):1536-1544. doi: 10.1016/j.jacc.2016.12.039.

[18] Brandt K, McGinn K, Quedado J. Low-Dose Systemic Alteplase (tPA) for the Treatment of Pulmonary Embolism. Ann Pharmacother. 2015 Jul;49(7):818-824.

[19] T. Capstick, M. T. Henry. Efficacy of thrombolytic agents in the treatment of pulmonary embolism. Eur Respir J. 2005;26:864-874; doi: 10.1183/09031936.05.00002505.

[20] Kiran GR, Chandrasekhar P, Ali SM. Association between 2D echocardiographic right atrial volume to left atrial volume (RAV/LAV) ratio and in-hospital prognosis in thrombolysed acute pulmonary thromboembolism patients. Indian Heart J. 2020;72(6): 610-613. doi:10.1016/j.ihj.2020.09.008.

[21] Roy PM, Douillet D, Penaloza A. Contemporary management of acute pulmonary embolism. Trends Cardiovasc Med. 2021 Jun 29:S1050-1738(21)00068-2. doi: 10.1016/j.tcm.2021.06.002.

[22] Pinede L, Duhaut P, Cucherat M, et al. Comparison of long versus short duration of anticoagulant therapy after a first episode of venous thromboembolism: a meta-analysis of randomized, controlled trials. J Intern Med. 2000 May;247(5):553-562. doi: 10.1046/j.1365-2796.2000.00631.x.

[23] de Winter MA, Vlachojannis GJ, Ruigrok D, Nijkeuter M, Kraaijeveld AO. Rationale for catheter-based therapies in acute pulmonary embolism. Eur Heart J Suppl. 2019 Nov;21(Suppl I): I16-I22. doi: 10.1093/eurheartj/suz223.

[24] Aggarwal V, Giri J, Nallamothu BK. Catheter-Based Therapies in Acute Pulmonary Embolism: The Good, the Bad, and the Ugly. Circ Cardiovasc Interv. 2020 Jun;13(6):e009353. doi: 10.1161/CIRCINTERVENTIONS. 120.009353.

[25] Avgerinos ED, Saadeddin Z, Abou Ali AN, et al. A meta-analysis of outcomes of catheter-directed thrombolysis for high- and intermediate-risk pulmonary embolism. J Vasc Surg Venous Lymphat Disord. 2018 Jul;6(4):530-540. doi: 10.1016/j.jvsv.2018.03.010.

[26] Rothschild DP, Goldstein JA, Ciacci J, et al. Ultrasound-accelerated thrombolysis (USAT) versus standard catheter-directed thrombolysis (CDT) for treatment of pulmonary embolism: A retrospective analysis. Vasc Med. 2019 Jun;24(3):234-240. doi: 10.1177/1358863X19838350.

[27] Rao G, Xu H, Wang JJ, Galmer A, et al. Ultrasound-assisted versus conventional catheter-directed thrombolysis for acute pulmonary embolism: A multicenter comparison of patient-centered outcomes. Vasc Med. 2019 Jun;24(3):241-247. doi: 10.1177/1358863X19838334.

[28] Avgerinos ED, Jaber W, Lacomis J, et al; SUNSET sPE Collaborators. Randomized Trial Comparing Standard Versus Ultrasound-Assisted Thrombolysis for Submassive Pulmonary Embolism: The SUNSET sPE Trial. JACC Cardiovasc Interv. 2021 Jun

28;14(12):1364-1373. doi: 10.1016/j. jcin.2021.04.049

[29] Pei DT, Liu J, Yaqoob M, et al. Meta-Analysis of Catheter Directed Ultrasound-Assisted Thrombolysis in Pulmonary Embolism. Am J Cardiol. 2019 Nov 1;124(9):1470-1477. doi: 10.1016/j.amjcard.2019.07.040.

[30] Siordia JA, Kaur A. Catheter-Directed Thrombolysis versus Systemic Anticoagulation for Submassive Pulmonary Embolism: A Meta-Analysis. Curr Cardiol Rev. 2021 Jun 3. doi: 10.217 4/1573403X17666210603114116.

[31] Hobohm L, Schmidt FP, Gori T, et al. In-hospital outcomes of catheter-directed thrombolysis in patients with pulmonary embolism. Eur Heart J Acute Cardiovasc Care. 2021 May 11;10(3):258-264. doi: 10.1093/ehjacc/ zuaa026.

[32] Chopard R, Ecarnot F, Meneveau N. Catheter-directed therapy for acute pulmonary embolism: navigating gaps in the evidence. Eur Heart J Suppl. 2019 Nov;21(Suppl I):I23-I30. doi: 10.1093/ eurheartj/suz224.

[33] Loyalka P, Ansari MZ, Cheema FH, et al. Surgical pulmonary embolectomy and catheter-based therapies for acute pulmonary embolism: A contemporary systematic review. J Thorac Cardiovasc Surg. 2018 Dec;156(6):2155-2167. doi: 10.1016/j.jtcvs.2018.05.085.

[34] Kalra R, Bajaj NS, Arora P, et al. Surgical Embolectomy for Acute Pulmonary Embolism: Systematic Review and Comprehensive Meta-Analyses. Ann Thorac Surg. 2017 Mar;103(3):982-990. doi: 10.1016/j. athoracsur.2016.11.016.

[35] D'Agostino C, Zonzin P, Enea I et al. ANMCO Position paper: long-term follow-up of patients with pulmonary thromboembolism. Eur Heart J. 2017;19(Suppl D):D309-32. doi: 10.1093/ eurheartj/sux030.

[36] Den Exter PL, van Es J, Kroft LJ, et al; Prometheus Follow-Up Investigators. Thromboembolic resolution assessed by CT pulmonary angiography after treatment for acute pulmonary embolism. Thromb Haemost. 2015 Jul;114(1):26-34. doi: 10.1160/TH14-10-0842. Epub 2015 May 28.

[37] Kabrhel C, Rosovsky R, Baugh C, et al. The creation and implementation of an outpatient pulmonary embolism treatment protocol. Hosp Pract (1995). 2017 Aug;45(3):123-129. doi: 10.1080/21548331.2017.1318651.

[38] Stern RM, Al-Samkari H, Connors JM. Thrombophilia evaluation in pulmonary embolism. Curr Opin Cardiol. 2019 Nov;34(6):603-609. doi: 10.1097/HCO.0000000000000668.

[39] Elsebaie MAT, van Es N, Langston A, et al. Direct oral anticoagulants in patients with venous thromboembolism and thrombophilia: a systematic review and meta-analysis. J Thromb Haemost. 2019 Apr;17(4): 645-656. doi: 10.1111/jth.14398.

[40] Marín-Romero S, Jara-Palomares L. Screening for occult cancer: where are we in 2020? Thromb Res. 2020 Jul;191 Suppl 1:S12-S16. doi: 10.1016/ S0049-3848(20)30390-X

[41] Ihaddadene R, Corsi DJ, Lazo-Langner A, et al. Risk factors predictive of occult cancer detection in patients with unprovoked venous thromboembolism. Blood. 2016;127(16):2035-2037. doi:10.1182/ blood-2015-11-682963.

[42] Kunutsor SK, Seidu S, Khunti K. Statins and primary prevention of venous thromboembolism: a systematic review and meta-analysis. Lancet Haematol. 2017 Feb;4(2):e83-e93. doi: 10.1016/S2352-3026(16)30184-3.

[43] Li R, Yuan M, Yu S, et al. Effect of statins on the risk of recurrent venous

thromboembolism: A systematic review and meta-analysis. Pharmacol Res. 2021 Mar;165:105413. doi: 10.1016/j. phrs.2020.105413.

[44] Key NS, Khorana AA, Kuderer NM, et al. Venous Thromboembolism Prophylaxis and Treatment in Patients With Cancer: ASCO Clinical Practice Guideline Update. J Clin Oncol. 2020 Feb 10;38(5):496-520. doi: 10.1200/ JCO.19.01461.

[45] Nicholson M, Chan N, Bhagirath V, Ginsberg J. Prevention of Venous Thromboembolism in 2020 and Beyond. J Clin Med. 2020 Aug 1;9(8):2467. doi: 10.3390/jcm9082467.

[46] DeYoung E, Minocha J. Inferior Vena Cava Filters: Guidelines, Best Practice, and Expanding Indications. Semin Intervent Radiol. 2016;33(2): 65-70. doi:10.1055/s-0036-1581088.

[47] Desai MM, Bracken MB, Spencer FA, et al. Inferior Vena Cava Filters to Prevent Pulmonary Embolism: Systematic Review and Meta-Analysis. J Am Coll Cardiol. 2017 Sep 26;70(13):1587-1597. doi: 10.1016/j. jacc.2017.07.775.

[48] Bikdeli B, Jiménez D, Kirtane AJ, et al. Systematic review of efficacy and safety of retrievable inferior vena caval filters. Thromb Res. 2018;165:79-82. doi:10.1016/j. thromres.2018.03.014.

[49] Deso SE, Idakoji IA, Kuo WT. Evidence-Based Evaluation of Inferior Vena Cava Filter Complications Based on Filter Type. Semin Intervent Radiol. 2016 Jun;33(2):93-100. doi: 10.1055/s-0036-1583208

[50] Yoo HH, Nunes-Nogueira VS, Fortes Villas Boas PJ. Anticoagulant treatment for subsegmental pulmonary embolism. Cochrane Database Syst Rev. 2020 Feb 7;2(2):CD010222. doi: 10.1002/14651858. CD010222.pub4.

[51] Donato AA, Khoche S, Santora J, Wagner B. Clinical outcomes in patients with isolated subsegmental pulmonary emboli diagnosed by multidetector CT pulmonary angiography. Thromb Res. 2010 Oct;126(4):e266-70. doi: 10.1016/j. thromres.2010.07.001.

[52] Carrier M, Klok FA. Symptomatic subsegmental pulmonary embolism: to treat or not to treat?. Hematology Am Soc Hematol Educ Program. 2017;2017(1):237-241. doi:10.1182/ asheducation-2017.1.237.

[53] Baumgartner, C, Tritschler, T. Clinical significance of subsegmental pulmonary embolism: An ongoing controversy. Res Pract Thromb Haemost. 2021; 5: 14– 16. https://doi. org/10.1002/rth2.12464.

[54] Newnham M, Turner AM. Diagnosis and treatment of subsegmental pulmonary embolism. World J Respirol 2019; 9(3): 30-34. doi: 10.5320/wjr. v9.i3.30.

[55] Suh YJ, Hong H, Ohana M, et al. Pulmonary Embolism and Deep Vein Thrombosis in COVID-19: A Systematic Review and Meta-Analysis. Radiology. 2021 Feb;298(2):E70-E80. doi: 10.1148/ radiol.2020203557.

[56] Roncon L, Zuin M, Barco S, et al. Incidence of acute pulmonary embolism in COVID-19 patients: Systematic review and meta-analysis. Eur J Intern Med. 2020 Dec;82:29-37. doi: 10.1016/j. ejim.2020.09.006.

[57] Kwee RM, Adams HJA, Kwee TC. Pulmonary embolism in patients with COVID-19 and value of D-dimer assessment: a meta-analysis. Eur Radiol. 2021 May 9:1-19. doi: 10.1007/ s00330-021-08003-8.

[58] Rico-Mesa JS, Rosas D, Ahmadian-Tehrani A, White A, Anderson AS, Chilton R. The Role of Anticoagulation in COVID-19-Induced

Hypercoagulability. Curr Cardiol Rep. 2020 Jun 17;22(7):53. doi: 10.1007/s11886-020-01328-8.

[59] McBane RD 2nd, Torres Roldan VD, Niven AS, et al. Anticoagulation in COVID-19: A Systematic Review, Meta-analysis, and Rapid Guidance From Mayo Clinic. Mayo Clin Proc. 2020;95(11):2467-2486. doi:10.1016/j.mayocp.2020.08.030.

[60] Tassiopoulos AK, Mofakham S, Rubano JA, et al. D-Dimer-Driven Anticoagulation Reduces Mortality in Intubated COVID-19 Patients: A Cohort Study With a Propensity-Matched Analysis. Front. Med. 8:631335. doi: 10.3389/fmed.2021.631335.

[61] Chandra A, Chakraborty U, Ghosh S, Dasgupta S. Anticoagulation in COVID-19: current concepts and controversies. Postgrad Med J. 2021 Apr 13: postgradmedj-2021-139923. doi: 10.1136/postgradmedj-2021-139923.

[62] Kaptein FHJ, Stals MAM, Huisman MV, Klok FA. Prophylaxis and treatment of COVID-19 related venous thromboembolism. Postgrad Med. 2021 Mar 4:1-9. doi: 10.1080/00325481.2021.1891788.

[63] Oudkerk M, Büller HR, Kuijpers D, et al. Diagnosis, Prevention, and Treatment of Thromboembolic Complications in COVID-19: Report of the National Institute for Public Health of the Netherlands. Radiology. 2020 Oct;297(1):E216-E222. doi: 10.1148/radiol.2020201629.

[64] Carfora V, Spiniello G, Ricciolino R, et al. Vanvitelli COVID-19 group. Anticoagulant treatment in COVID-19: a narrative review. J Thromb Thrombolysis. 2021 Apr;51(3):642-648. doi: 10.1007/s11239-020-02242-0.

[65] Asakura, H., Ogawa, H. Perspective on fibrinolytic therapy in COVID-19: the potential of inhalation therapy against suppressed-fibrinolytic-type DIC. j intensive care 8, 71 (2020). https://doi.org/10.1186/s40560-020-00491-y.

[66] Hsieh WC, Jansa P, Huang WC, et al. Residual pulmonary hypertension after pulmonary endarterectomy: A meta-analysis. J Thorac Cardiovasc Surg. 2018 Sep;156(3):1275-1287. doi: 10.1016/j.jtcvs.2018.04.110.

[67] Kalra R, Duval S, Thenappan T, et al. Comparison of Balloon Pulmonary Angioplasty and Pulmonary Vasodilators for Inoperable Chronic Thromboembolic Pulmonary Hypertension: A Systematic Review and Meta-Analysis. Sci Rep. 2020 Jun 1;10(1):8870. doi: 10.1038/s41598-020-65697-4.

[68] Phan K, Jo HE, Xu J, Lau EM. Medical Therapy Versus Balloon Angioplasty for CTEPH: A Systematic Review and Meta-Analysis. Heart Lung Circ. 2018 Jan;27(1):89-98. doi: 10.1016/j.hlc.2017.01.016. Epub 2017 Mar 1.

[69] Khan MS, Amin E, et al. Meta-analysis of use of balloon pulmonary angioplasty in patients with inoperable chronic thromboembolic pulmonary hypertension. Int J Cardiol. 2019 Sep 15;291:134-139. doi: 10.1016/j.ijcard.2019.02.051. Epub 2019 Feb 23.

[70] Bunclark K, Newnham M, Chiu YD, et al. A multicenter study of anticoagulation in operable chronic thromboembolic pulmonary hypertension. J Thromb Haemost. 2020 Jan;18(1):114-122. doi: 10.1111/jth.14649.

[71] Gavilanes-Oleas FA, Alves JL Jr, Fernandes CJC, et al. Use of direct oral anticoagulants for chronic thromboembolic pulmonary hypertension. *Clinics (Sao Paulo).* 2018;73:e216. Published 2018 May 17. doi:10.6061/clinics/2018/e216.

[72] Papamatheakis DG, Poch DS, Fernandes TM, Kerr KM, Kim NH, Fedullo PF. Chronic Thromboembolic Pulmonary Hypertension: JACC Focus Seminar. J Am Coll Cardiol. 2020 Nov 3;76(18):2155-2169. doi: 10.1016/j. jacc.2020.08.074. PMID: 33121723.

[73] hang L, Bai Y, Yan P, He T, et al. Balloon pulmonary angioplasty vs. pulmonary endarterectomy in patients with chronic thromboembolic pulmonary hypertension: a systematic review and meta-analysis. Heart Fail Rev. 2021 Feb 5. doi: 10.1007/ s10741-020-10070-w.

[74] Rivera-Lebron B, McDaniel M, Ahrar K, PERT Consortium et al. Diagnosis, treatment and follow up of acute pulmonary embolism: consensus practice from the PERT Consortium. Clin Appl Thromb Hemost. 2019;25:1076029619853037. doi: 10.1177/1076029619853037

[75] Konstantinides SV, Meyer G, Becattini C, et al. ESC Scientific Document Group. 2019 ESC Guidelines for the diagnosis and management of acute pulmonary embolism developed in collaboration with the European Respiratory Society (ERS). Eur Heart J. 2020 Jan 21;41(4):543-603. doi: 10.1093/ eurheartj/ehz405.

[76] Ortel TL, Neumann I, Ageno W, et al. American Society of Hematology 2020 guidelines for management of venous thromboembolism: treatment of deep vein thrombosis and pulmonary embolism. Blood Adv. 2020 Oct 13;4(19):4693-4738. doi: 10.1182/ bloodadvances.2020001830

[77] Giri J, Sista AK, Weinberg I, et al. Interventional Therapies for Acute Pulmonary Embolism: Current Status and Principles for the Development of Novel Evidence: A Scientific Statement From the American Heart Association. Circulation. 2019 Nov 12;140(20):

e774-e801. doi: 10.1161/CIR. 0000000000000707. Epub 2019 Oct 4. PMID: 31585051.

[78] Duranteau J, Taccone FS, Verhamme P, et al; ESA VTE Guidelines Task Force. European guidelines on perioperative venous thromboembolism prophylaxis: Intensive care. Eur J Anaesthesiol. 2018 Feb;35(2):142-146. doi: 10.1097/EJA.0000000000000707. PMID: 29112545.

[79] Key NS, Khorana AA, Kuderer NM, et al. Venous Thromboembolism Prophylaxis and Treatment in Patients With Cancer: ASCO Clinical Practice Guideline Update. J Clin Oncol. 2020 Feb 10;38(5):496-520. doi: 10.1200/ JCO.19.01461.

[80] Delcroix M, Torbicki A, Gopalan D, et al. ERS Statement on Chronic Thromboembolic Pulmonary Hypertension. Eur Respir J. 2020 Dec 17:2002828. doi: 10.1183/ 13993003.02828-2020

[81] Kaufman JA, Barnes GD, Chaer RA, et al. Society of Interventional Radiology Clinical Practice Guideline for Inferior Vena Cava Filters in the Treatment of Patients with Venous Thromboembolic Disease: Developed in collaboration with the American College of Cardiology, American College of Chest Physicians, American College of Surgeons Committee on Trauma, American Heart Association, Society for Vascular Surgery, and Society for Vascular Medicine. J Vasc Interv Radiol. 2020 Oct;31(10):1529-1544. doi: 10.1016/j.jvir.2020.06.014.

[82] Cuker A, Tseng EK, Nieuwlaat R, et al. American Society of Hematology 2021 guidelines on the use of anticoagulation for thromboprophylaxis in patients with COVID-19. Blood Adv. 2021 Feb 9;5(3):872-888. doi: 10.1182/ bloodadvances.2020003763.

Chapter 8

Advances of Thrombectomy in Venous Thromboembolism

Jia-Ling Lin, Po-Sheng Chen, Po-Kai Yang and Chih-Hsin Hsu

Abstract

Venous thromboembolism (VTE) presenting as deep vein thrombosis and pulmonary embolism clinically is a potentially fatal cardiovascular diseases with short-term and long-term sequelae. Furthermore, there is high recurrent rate in VTE patients during follow-up. Anticoagulation with traditional anticoagulants or new generation of oral anticoagulants is the gold standard treatment in patients with VTE. On the other hand, there is remarkable progression in device-based or surgical thrombectomy in managements of VTE in recent years. Current evidence also demonstrates the efficacy and safety of these invasive procedures in selective VTE patients. The present article will illustrate recent advances of device-based or surgical thrombectomy in VTE treatment.

Keywords: deep vein thrombosis, pulmonary embolism, catheter-directed thrombolysis, (mechanical thrombectomy), rheolytic embolectomy, aspiration thrombectomy, rotational thrombectomy

1. Introduction

Venous thromboembolism (VTE) is a set of diseases in which blood clot forms and occludes venous circulation and regard as the third frequent acute cardio-vascular disease [1]. Clinically, VTE presents as deep vein thrombosis (DVT) and pulmonary embolism (PE) which account for two-third and one-third of VTE, respectively [2]. The estimated annual rate of incidence of VTE is 80 to 260 per 100000 population [3]. In general, the incidence of VTE increases with age. One epidemiologic study in United States showed that the incidence of VTE was 143 per 100000 in papulation at age 45–49 years and 1134 per 100000 in those at age > 80 years [4]. There is difference of incidence between ethnicities and black and white have higher incidence than other races [2]. Although patients with VTE might be asymptomatic, VTE is a potentially fatal disease. One study reported that the estimated annual VTE-related death was around 300000 in U.S [5] and nearly 30% of VTE patients died within 30 days after diagnosis. Compared to DVT, PE accounts for majority of early-stage mortality of VTE [6, 7]. In addition to VTE-related mortality and cardiovascular sequelae, such as post-thrombotic syndrome, chronic venous insufficiency and chronic thromboembolic pulmonary hyperten-sion, etc., patients with VTE have high risk of other atherosclerotic diseases and acute cardiovascular events, such as acute myocardial infarction and ischemic stroke, in the short-term and long-term follow-up [8–10]. With a brief review of pathogenesis and risk factors of VTE, the following of this chapter focuses on percutaneous interventions for VTE.

2. Pathogenesis and risk factors of venous thromboembolism

Virchow's triad composed of stasis, vascular damage and hypercoagulable status describes the essential components contributing to the thrombus formation [11]. In most cases of VTE, stasis plays a major role triggering the formation of venous thrombosis [12]. However, the exact pathogenesis of VTE seems to be more complex and is not fully understood [2, 13]. Only one existing contributing factor is hard to result in the development of clot formation [14]. Nonetheless, the interaction between multiple concurrent contributing factors increases the risk of formation of venous thrombosis which progresses to significant VTE clinically thereafter.

In clinical aspect, many diseases and circumstances regarded as risk factors are identified to predispose to the development of VTE. In general, these risk factors are classified into genetic and acquired risk [15–18]. Genetic risk factors including protein C and S deficiency, antithrombin deficiency, the factor V Leiden gene mutation, antiphospholipid syndrome, etc. Acquired risk factors are further divided into concurrent diseases (elderly, chronic diseases, active cancer, obesity) and transient states (surgery, trauma, hospitalization, immobility, central venous catheter or device indwelling, oral contraceptives, etc.) [2]. Of note, hospitalization is an important period that multiple risk factors encounter concurrently and increase the risk of VTE greatly [2, 19]. Although predisposing factors are identified in most cases of VTE, there are still almost 20% of case having no obvious etiology. The result suggests the significance of unknown genetic or acquired risk factors to the development of VTE [2, 3].

3. Thrombectomy in management of VTE

To date, anticoagulation is still the principal treatment in VTE. In addition to traditional anticoagulation, including heparin, low molecular weight heparin and vitamin K antagonists, as well as direct thrombin inhibitors, non-vitamin K oral anticoagulants (NOACs), known as direct oral-anticoagulant (DOACs) change the strategy in medical treatment of VTE. The update of principles and strategies of medical treatment of VTM will be illustrated in another chapter. On the other hand, endovascular or surgical thrombectomy and embolectomy have role in treatment of VTE. Historically, Läwen conducted the first thrombectomy for venous thrombosis of upper extremity in 1938 [20]. After evolution in nearly 90 years, there are great advances in techniques and modalities in performing thrombectomy and embolectomy. However, thrombectomy or embolectomy is still indicated in limited population in modern treatment of VTE, especially in patients with massive or submassive thrombus burden accompanied by unstable hemodynamic status or critical complications [21–23]. Theoretically, endovascular or surgical thrombectomy removes majority of thrombus load more completely and recanalization of occluded vessels earlier [24, 25]. Moreover, some previous studies even reported that thrombectomy may have potential benefits comparing to anticoagulation alone in long-term complications and quality of life in certain VTE patients [22, 26]. The aim of this chapter will focus on the advances of modalities of endovascular and surgical thrombectomy.

4. Catheter-based therapy

Percutaneous management, also known as catheter-based therapy (CBT), for VTE can be divided into two mechanisms: thrombolysis-based and mechanical thrombectomy. There are also devices combining these two mechanisms. For certain conditions, percutaneous approaches also include balloon angioplasty and stenting. We describe different types of CBT in the following sections.

4.1 Catheter-directed thrombolysis

Compared to systemic thrombolysis, catheter-based thrombolysis is, by concept, more likely a local therapy. The advantage of this approach is a reduced-dose thrombolysis. Therefore, there is less risk of bleeding [27, 28]. Although with lower dosage needed, absolute contraindications for catheter-directed thrombolysis are the same as for systemic thrombolysis, including history of any intracranial hemorrhage, ischemic stroke within three months, structural intra-cranial lesion, active bleeding, recent head, eye or spinal surgery, and recent head trauma [29, 30].

This approach is done by placing an infusion catheter with multiple side holes and a tip occluding wire or a dedicated catheter specifically for a certain device, preferentially into the thrombus. It may sometimes require two catheters to be placed in each of the main pulmonary arteries. If there is no specialized catheter, a standard pig-tail or pulmonary artery catheter may also serve to deliver thrombo-lytic agent locally. When performing intervention for pulmonary embolism (PE), power injection may be necessary to take clear angiography to localizes the emboli. For each main pulmonary artery, perform contrast injection at 15–20 m/s for a total volume of 30 ml [28]. For intervention of deep venous thrombosis (DVT), careful hand injection with low-volume contrast is preferred to avoid disruption of thrombi with progression to PE [30].

Thrombolytic agent is administered via the carefully placed catheter. There is no standard for the agent and dosage used. It varies according to accompanied device, patients' bleeding tendency, and physicians' preferences. A commonly used regimen is tissue plasminogen activator (tPA) 0.5–1.0 mg/hr for 6–24 hours, with total dosage usually between 12 and 24 mg. Fibrinogen should be monitored during infusion of fibrinolytic agent. Dose reduction or discontinuation should be consid-ered if level of fibrinogen falls below 150 mg/dL. During t-PA infusion, a low-dose heparin infusion is usually kept, with a partial thromboplastin time (PTT) just around the lower limit of therapeutic range, usually PTT 40–50 seconds [28, 30].

Catheter-directed thrombolysis applies for both DVT and PE. A key factor to success of lytic-based approach is that whether the thrombolytic agent is delivered into the thrombus with good penetration. A resolution to this problem is combining other method to enhance efficacy of drug delivery, such as the EkoSonic system.

EkoSonic™ Endovascular System (EKOS) is a device for ultrasound-assisted catheter-directed thrombolysis. It includes a control unit and a uniquely designed catheter to achieve better penetration of thrombolytics by so-called acoustic pulse thrombolysis. The catheter is composed of an ultrasonic core in central lumen, central coolant lumen, and drug delivery lumen. The ultrasonic core generates an acoustic field to enhance drug delivery into the clot and to unwind the fibrin for better exposure to thrombolytic agents. This system is indicated for both DVT and PE [31].

There were also devices designed for a true localized therapy. Trellis™ Peripheral Infusion System is a specialized device for isolated thrombolysis. It consists of two occlusive balloons to isolate the treatment area, an infusion zone to deliver throm-bolytic agents, an oscillation drive unit to better disperse the drug to thrombi, and an aspiration window to remove the dissolved clot. Although with a unique design to ensure localized thrombolysis and thrombi removal, the devices were recalled due to incorrectly labelling of proximal and distal balloons [32].

Of note, catheter-directed thrombolysis alone may not be sufficient to clear all blood clots, although it is true that the goal of catheter-directed thrombolysis for PE is not to remove emboli completely, but to reduce the risk from high to intermediate [29]. Further intervention to remove emboli and thrombi may be needed and there are devices combining local thrombolysis and sequential blood clot removal, which would be described later.

4.2 Mechanical thrombectomy

Mechanical thrombectomy is achieved by physical disruption of thrombus via different methods, with various devices designed for this purpose. These devices have different benefits, adverse effects, and special concerns while manipulation. Overall, they are less invasive compared with traditional surgical thrombectomy. Some devices achieve thrombus removal in a single session, sparing the use of thrombolytic agents. The following section describes devices with approval. Devices still under development are not covered.

4.2.1 Thrombus fragmentation

Mechanical thrombectomy without a device has long been described in both treatment for DVT and PE. It is usually done by a pigtail with manual rotation or by balloon angioplasty [28]. An important issue of fragmentation is that it might create distal emboli, causing worse distal obstruction; and fragmentation alone may not be enough to resolve obstruction. It may be followed by systemic thrombolysis, catheter-directed thrombolysis, or thrombi removal by manual aspiration. Due to lack of clinical evidence, there is no recommendation for how to combine other strategy after manual thrombus fragmentation.

4.2.2 Aspiration thrombectomy

Besides manual thrombus aspiration with a regular guide catheter or specialized catheters with greater power of suction, there are devices designed to remove thrombus by suction via negative pressure. The advantages are the ability to remove large thrombi or even chronic thrombi, avoidance of thrombolytic agents, and possible less risk of bleeding.

The AngioVac® system works in an extracorporeal circuit and needs two large venous access sites for AngioVac inflow cannula (22Fr) and reinfusion outflow cannula (16–20 Fr). The third generation uses funnel-shaped and different-angled tip (20 degree or 180 degree) to facilitate navigation. Besides the need of two large-bore accesses, another disadvantage of this device is that perfusionist is required. It is indicated for removal of fresh, soft thrombi or emboli in right atrium, right ventricle, superior vena cava, inferior vena cava, and iliofemoral veins during extracorporeal bypass. It is not indicated in pulmonary vasculature although there are case series [33].

The FlowTriever® system includes an Triever Aspiration Catheter, a FlowTriever catheter, and a retraction aspiration device. Thrombus removal is done by manual aspiration with a syringe via the large-lumen aspiration catheter. There are nitinol mesh disks on the tip of FlowTriever catheter to disrupt and drag residual clots into the aspiration catheter for extraction. This system is indicated for PE [34]. A similar system dedicated for DVT is the ClotTriever® system. It includes a ClotTriever sheath and a ClotTriever catheter. The procedure steps are somewhat different. The ClotTriever catheter is position beyond the thrombus. A mesh collection bag on the tip of ClotTriever catheter retracts thrombi into the ClotTriever sheath with a self-expanding funnel tip, providing embolic protection. Manual aspiration is applied if there are residual thrombi in the sheath. Since treatment is completed in a single session and there is no need for thrombolysis, care in intensive care unit (ICU) after procedure may not be necessary. However, a large-bore vascular access (20 Fr) is needed [35].

Penumbra's Indigo® Aspiration System operates in a more "automatic" way, with less need of manual control. The main components of the system are a catheter, a Penumbra ENGINE to generate vacuum for aspiration, and a tubing system. When the catheter is in position, the system performs automatic aspiration. With different catheters, there are corresponding Separator wires to remove clot in the lumen of aspiration catheters. Compared to AngioVac® and FlowTriever®, the Indigo® system does not require large-bore vascular access but may therefore unable to remove larger thrombi. It is indicated for removal of fresh, soft thrombi or emboli in both peripheral arterial and venous system and for treatment of PE [36].

Syringed-based thrombectomy offers limited force and aspirated volume, and operators could not further manipulate. Pump systems with specific devices provide increased force and volume but usually with increased complexity of the procedure and increased cost. Control Mechanical Thrombectomy™ system (Aspire) works in a different way. The system includes a thrombectomy catheter and a control mechanical aspirator which is like a handle. Through the handle, the operator can adjust strength of the aspirated force, and switch between continuous and pulsed force. It is indicated for removal of fresh, soft thrombi in peripheral vasculature, but not PE [37].

4.2.3 Rotational thrombectomy

The concept of rotational thrombectomy is thrombus disruption by a catheter with rotating head. Most devices also have the ability to remove thrombus via active suction.

Aspirex® mechanical thrombectomy device consists of a catheter with a handle and a drive system. At the tip of the catheter, there is aspiration port to suck in thrombi; and inside the catheter, there is rotational coil to break down thrombi. The fragmented thrombi are then aspirated out. The device is indicated for both arterial and venous thrombi. With limited case studies, it is not approved for treatment of PE [38].

CLEANER™ Rotational Thrombectomy System is a one-piece device. Rotating action of its sinusoidal wire breaks down thrombi. The sinusoidal shape provides atraumatic action on thrombi adhered to vessel wall. The device also enables infusion of thrombolytic agents via a distal side hole. It is indicated for removal of thrombus in peripheral vasculature, but not for PE [39].

4.2.4 Rheolytic thrombectomy

Rheolytic thrombectomy is based on Bernoulli effect. A high-velocity saline jet creates a low-pressure, drawing thrombi into the catheter. To eliminate thrombi better, it may be accompanied with thrombolysis or other mechanical method such as aspiration.

Among this category, the mostly studied device is AngioJet™ Rheolytic Thrombectomy System, consisting of a console and a thrombectomy catheter. The system works in both pharmacological and mechanical ways. Operators can deliver thrombolytic agents directly into the clot to facilitate removal of thrombus. The console generates pressurized saline to draw thrombi into the catheter via an inflow window near the tip of the catheter, and then evacuates the thrombi.

Notable adverse events include pain, cardiac arrythmia (mainly bradyarrhythmia), hypotension, transient hemolysis, bleeding, and acute kidney injury. Hydration before, during, and after the procedure may be considered. AngioJet™ system is indicated in removal of thrombi in peripheral vasculature. When used in PE, there were severe adverse events, including death; so, there is a "black box" warning for AngioJet™ in treating PE [40].

4.3 Combined thrombolytic and mechanical approaches

The concept of combination works in at least two modes. One is to combine multiple mechanisms at the same time, usually by devices, like EKOS or AngioJet™. The other way is to use different methods sequentially. For instance, physicians may perform balloon angioplasty first to disrupt the thrombi; and then leave an infusion catheter for thrombolysis. This concept also works in a reverse way. Physicians may place an infusion catheter for thrombolysis first, usually for 24 hours; and then break the loosen thrombi with balloon angioplasty. Theoretically, combing thrombolysis and mechanical thrombectomy improves efficacy of thrombus removal, but there is no standard for how to combine multiple strategies due to limited studies. This so-called pharmacomechanical approach is therefore, largely based on clinicians' experience.

4.4 Angioplasty and stenting

Besides thrombolysis and mechanical thrombectomy, some adjuvant procedures may be needed, mainly for DVT. Balloon angioplasty plays a role in chronic thromboembolic pulmonary hypertension, but not for acute PE. For DVT, placement of inferior vena cava filter before procedure may be considered to prevent PE, especially for patients with poor cardiopulmonary function and deemed unable to tolerate PE [30]. The results of studies regarding stenting for DVT were inconsistent, although some showed reduced severity in post-thrombotic syndrome and improved quality of life in some aspects [41–43]. This approach is therefore largely based on clinicians' experience.

Stenting is considered if there is residual thrombi or residual venous outflow obstruction. It may also be considered when there is non-thrombotic cause of stenosis, such as in May-Thurner syndrome. Therefore, careful assessment of the lesion is important. It is helpful to combine other image modality such as computed tomography or intravascular ultrasound. Besides anatomical nature, clinicians should put patients' life expectancy, bleeding risk, and likelihood of symptom improvement into consideration. When a stent is placed, there is always risk of in-stent restenosis or occlusion. Risk factors include poor inflow, external compression, inappropriate stent design, stent misplacement or migration, stent fracture, and bleeding. Patients should be notified about the possibility of reintervention [44].

4.5 Summary of catheter-based therapy

The purpose of CBT is to relieve obstruction quicker, compared with traditional medical therapy. However, there is no strong evidence that CBT is better than traditional systemic thrombolysis since randomized trial assessing hard outcomes, such as mortality, is lacking. Also, among CBT, there is no trial comparing catheter-directed thrombolysis and mechanical thrombectomy or comparing different devices. It is also important to remember that published studies for CBT with devices are of small patient numbers. There are many trials still going on. Hopefully, these trials will provide evidences for more specific guidance.

For any intervention, there are always complications. Possible complications of CBT include access site bleeding, vascular injury, major bleeding (including intracranial hemorrhage), distal emboli (especially of concern with PE when performing intervention for DVT), cardiac tamponade (intervention for PE), hemodynamic deterioration, and deterioration in renal function. Some studies did not demonstrate the presumed benefit of less major bleedings (including intracranial hemorrhage) in percutaneous methods, compared with systemic thrombolysis [28, 29]. The balance between risk and benefit of these interventions should be personalized.

Generally speaking, CBT may be considered in patients with iliofemoral DVT who have severe symptoms and a low risk of bleeding [45]. For PE, CBT is an alternative to systemic thrombolysis and surgical embolectomy, considered when these approaches are contraindicated or fail [46]. For now, the choice of CBT largely remains on physicians' experience and local availability.

5. Surgical embolectomy

Surgical intervention is an old skill compared with percutaneous intervention. Surgical embolectomy of PE requires cardiopulmonary bypass. After thoracotomy, emboli are removed manually with forceps. Balloon catheter and suction may be used for residual emboli. Although surgical embolectomy is a class I indication for massive pulmonary embolism, it is usually reserved as a salvage therapy when other therapies fail or are contraindicated, due to its invasive nature. If there is thrombus in right heart or thrombus across patent foramen ovale, surgical embolectomy would be considered the first-line therapy [27].

On the other hand, surgical thrombectomy for DVT is usually done with a special balloon catheter to pull out thrombi in the direction of venous flow, called Fogarty maneuvers [47]. Unlike for PE, surgical thrombectomy for DVT is not recommended by clinical guidelines. Although there are studies showing good patency rates after surgery, it is usually considered only in certain conditions when rapid reduction of venous obstruction is needed, such as in patients with phlegmasia cerulea dolens [48].

6. Conclusions

Although rapid evolution of modalities and relatively high successful rate in experienced center, routine use of endovascular or surgical thrombectomy and thrombolysis in patient with VTE is not recommended. To date, large-scale clinical trial assessing the efficacy and safety of invasive thrombolysis or thrombectomy is still lack. The application of endovascular or surgical strategies should be considered in selective VTE patients with unstable hemodynamic status or critical VTE-associated complications or having contraindications or high risk of bleeding while receiving systemic thrombolysis. In addition, future studies focusing on cost-effectiveness are needed to integrate these invasive procedures with medical strategies in the protocol of VTE treatment.

Author details

Jia-Ling Lin[1,2], Po-Sheng Chen[1,3], Po-Kai Yang[2] and Chih-Hsin Hsu[1,3*]

1 Division of Cardiology, Department of Internal Medicine, National Cheng Kung University Hospital, Tainan, Taiwan

2 Division of Cardiology, Department of Internal Medicine, National Cheng Kung University Hospital, Dou-Liou Branch, College of Medicine, National Cheng Kung University, Yunlin, Taiwan

3 Division of Critical Care, Department of Internal Medicine, National Cheng Kung University Hospital, College of Medicine, National Cheng Kung University, Tainan, Taiwan

*Address all correspondence to: chihhsinhsu@gmail.com

IntechOpen

References

[1] Raskob GE, Angchaisuksiri P, Blanco AN, et al. Thrombosis: a major contributor to global disease burden. Arterioscler Thromb Vasc Biol 2014;34:2363 2371. DOI: 10.1161/ATVBAHA.114.304488.

[2] Beckman MG, Hooper WC, Critchley SE, et al. Venous thromboembolism: a public health concern. Am J Prev Med 2010;38: S495-S501. DOI: 10.1016/j.amepre.2009.12.017.

[3] Wendelboe AM, Raskob GE. Global burden of thrombosis: epidemiologic aspects. Circ Res 2016;118:1340-1347. DOI: 10.1161/CIRCRESAHA.115.306841.

[4] Venous thromboembolism in adult hospitalizations – United States, 2007-2009. MMWR Morbid Moral Wkly Rep. 2012;61:401-404.

[5] Heit JA, Cohen AT, Anderson Jr FA, on behalf of the VTE Impact Assessment Group. Estimated annual number of incident and recurrent on-fatal and fatal venous thromboembolism (VTE) event in US. Blood 2005;106:910. DOI: 10.1182/blood.V106.11.910.910

[6] Hei JA, Silverstein MD, Mohr DN et al. The epidemiology of venous thromboembolism in the community. Thromb Haemost 2001;86:452-463.

[7] Cushman M, Rsai AW, White RH, et al. Deep vein thrombosis and pulmonary embolism in two cohort: the longitudinal investigation of thromboembolism etiology. Am J Med 2004;117:19-25. DOI: 10.1016/j.amjmed.2004.01.018.

[8] Sørensen HT, Horvath-Puho E, Søgaar KK et al. Arterial cardiovascular events, statins, low-dose aspirin and subsequent risk of venous thromboembolism: a population-based case-control study. J Thromb Haemost 2009;7:521-528. DOI: 10.1111/j.1538-7836.2009.03279.x.

[9] Sørensen HT, Horvath-Puho E, Pedersen L, et al. Venous thromboembolism and subsequent hospitalization due to acute arterial cardiovascular events: a 20-year cohort study. Lancet 2007;370:1773-1779. DOI: 10.1016/S0140-6736(07)61745-0.

[10] Becattini C, Vedovati MC, Ageno W, et al. Incidence of arterial cardiovascular events after venous thromboembolism; a systemic review and a meta-analysis. J Thromb Haemost 2010;8:891-897. DOI: 10.1111/j.1538-7836.2010.03777.x.

[11] Popuri RK, Vedantham S. The role of thrombolysis in the clinical management of deep vein thrombosis. Arterioscler Thromb Vasc Biol 2011;31:479-484. DOI: 10.1161/ATVBAHA.110.213413.

[12] Behravesh S, Hoang P, Nanda A, et al. Pathogenesis of thromboembolism and endovascular management. Thrombosis 2017;2017:3039713. DOI: 10.1155/2017/3039713.

[13] Suwanabol PA, Hoch JR. Venous thromboembolic disease. Surg Clin N Am 2013;93:983-995. DOI: 10.1016/j.suc.2013.05.003.

[14] Wessler S, Reimer SM, Sheps MC. Biologic assay of a thrombosis-inducing activity in human serum. J Appl Physiol 1595;14:943-946. DOI: 10.1152/jappl.1959.14.6.943.

[15] Anderson Jr FA, Spencer FA. Risk factors for venous thromboembolism. Circulation 2003;107:I9-I16. DOI: 10.1161/01.CIR.0000078469.07362.E6.

[16] Dowling NF, Austin H, Dilley A et al. The epidemiology of venous thromboembolism in Caucasians and

African-Americans: the GATE Study. J Thrombo Haemost 2003;1:80-87. DOI: 10.1046/j.1538-7836.2003.00031.x.

[17] Rosendaal FR. Venous thrombosis: a multicausal disease. Lancet 1999;353:1167-1173. DOI: 10.1016/s0140-6736(98)10266-0.

[18] Prandoni P. Acquired risk factors for venous thromboembolism in medical patients. Pathophysiol Haemost Thromb 2006;35:128-132. DOI: 10.1159/000093554.

[19] Spencer FA, Lessard D, Emery C, et al. Venous thromboembolism in the outpatient setting. Arch Intern Med 2007;167:1471-1475. DOI: 10.1001/archinte.167.14.1471.

[20] Galanaud JP, Laroche JP, Righini M. The history and historical treatments of deep vein thrombosis. J Thromb Haemost 2013;11:402-411. DOI: 10.1111/jth.12127

[21] Vedantham S, Thorpe PE, Cardella JF et al. Quality improvement guidelines for the treatment of lower extremity deep vein thrombosis with use of endovascular thrombus removal. J Vasc Inter Radiol 2006;17:435-447. DOI: 10.1097/01.RVI.0000197348.57762.15.

[22] Nosher JL, Patel A, Jagpal S, et al. Endovascular treatment of pulmonary embolism: selective review of available techniques. World J Radiol 2017;9:426-437. DOI: 10.4329/wjr.v9.i12.426

[23] Tice C, Seigerman M, Fiorlli P, et al. Management of acute pulmonary embolism. Curr Cardiovasc Risk Rep 2020;14:24. DOI: 10.1007/s12170-020-00659-z.

[24] Dudzinski DM, Giri J, Rosenfield K. Interventional treatment of pulmonary embolism. Circ Cardiovasc Interv 2017;10:e004345. DOI: 10.1161/CIRCINTERVENTIONS.116.004345

[25] Patterson B, Hinchliffe R, Loftus IM, et al. Indications for catheter-directed thrombolysis in the management of acute proximal deep venous thrombosis. Arterioscler Thromb Vasc Biol 2010;30:669-674. DOI: 10.1161/ATVBAHA.109.200766.

[26] Fleck D, Albadawi H, Shamoun F, et al. Catheter-directed thrombolysis of deep vein thrombosis: literature review and practice considerations. Cardiovasc Diagn Ther 2017;7: S228-S237. DOI: 10.21037/cdt.2017.09.15.

[27] Bernal AG, Fanonla C, Bartos JA. Management of PE expert analysis [Internet]. Jan 27, 2020. Available from: https://www.acc.org/latest-in-cardiology/articles/2020/01/27/07/42/management-of-pe [Accessed 2021-07-19]

[28] Jaber WA, Fong PP, Weisz G, et al. Acute pulmonary embolism: with an emphasis on an interventional approach. J Am Coll Cardiol 2016;67:991-1002. doi: 10.1016/j.jacc.2015.12.024.

[29] Giri J, Sista AK, Weinberg I, et al. Interventional therapies for acute pulmonary embolism: current status and principles for the development of novel evidence: a scientific statement from the American Heart Association. Circulation. 2019;140(20):e774-e801. doi: 10.1161/CIR.0000000000000707.

[30] Kohi MP, Kohlbrenner R, Kolli KP, Lehrman E, Taylor AG, Fidelman N. Catheter directed interventions for acute deep vein thrombosis. Cardiovasc Diagn Ther. 2016;6(6):599-611. doi: 10.21037/cdt.2016.11.20.

[31] EkoSonic™ Endovascular System [Internet]. 2021. Available from: https://www.bostonscientific.com/en-US/products/thrombectomy-systems/ekosonic-endovascular-system.html [Accessed 2021-07-25]

[32] Covidien Launches Next-Generation Trellis™ Peripheral Infusion System [Internet]. Jul 8, 2014. Available from: https://news.medtronic.com/2014-07-08-Covidien-Launches-Next-Generation-Trellis-TM-Peripheral-Infusion-System [Accessed 2021-07-25]

[33] AngioVac Cannula and Circuit Overview [Internet]. 2021. Available from: https://www.angiovac.com/overview-gen-3/ [Accessed 2021-07-25]

[34] FlowTriever® The First Mechanical Thrombectomy Device Indicated for Pulmonary Embolism [Internet]. 2021. Available from: https://www.inarimedical.com/int/flowtriever/ [Accessed 2021-07-25]

[35] ClotTriever® Extracting large clots from large vessels without the need for thrombolytics [Internet]. 2021. Available from: https://www.inarimedical.com/clottriever/ [Accessed 2021-07-25]

[36] Indigo System [Internet]. 2021. Available from: https://www.penumbrainc.com/de-ch/peripheral-device/indigo-system/ [Accessed 2021-07-25]

[37] CONTROL MECHANICAL THROMBECTOMY™ [Internet]. 2021. Available from: http://www.aspirationmedical.com/ [Accessed 2021-07-25]

[38] Straub Endovascular System [Internet]. 2021. https://pdf.medicalexpo.com/pdf/straub-medical/rotarex-s-aspirex-s/86437-109819.html#open583079 [Accessed 2021-07-25]

[39] CLEANER™ Rotational Thrombectomy System [Internet]. 2021. Available from: https://www.argonmedical.com/products/cleaner-rotational-thrombectomy-system [Accessed 2021-07-25]

[40] AngioJet™ Ultra Peripheral Thrombectomy System [Internet]. 2021. Available from: https://www.bostonscientific.com/en-EU/products/thrombectomy-systems/angiojet-thrombectomy-system.html [Accessed 2021-07-25]

[41] Vedantham S, Goldhaber SZ, Julian JA, et al. Pharmacomechanical catheter-directed thrombolysis for deep-vein thrombosis. N Engl J Med. 2017;377(23):2240-2252. DOI: 10.1056/NEJMoa1615066.

[42] Haig Y, Enden T, Grotta O, et al. Post-thrombotic syndrome after catheter-directed thrombolysis for deep vein thrombosis (CaVenT): 5-year follow-up results of an open-label, randomised controlled trial. Lancet Haematol. 2016;3(2):e64-e71. DOI: 10.1016/S2352-3026(15)00248-3.

[43] Comerota AJ, Kearon C, Gu CS, et al. Endovascular thrombus removal for acute iliofemoral deep vein thrombosis. Circulation. 2019;139(9):1162-1173. DOI: 10.1161/CIRCULATIONAHA.118.037425.

[44] Karen Breen. Role of venous stenting for venous thromboembolism. Hematology Am Soc Hematol Educ Program. 2020 Dec 4;2020(1):606-611. DOI: 10.1182/hematology.2020000147.

[45] Chopard R, Albertsen IE, Piazza G. Diagnosis and treatment of lower extremity venous thromboembolism: a review. JAMA. 2020;324(17):1765-1776. DOI:10.1001/jama.2020.17272.

[46] Konstantinides SV, Meyer G, Becattini C, et al. 2019 ESC Guidelines for the diagnosis and management of acute pulmonary embolism developed in collaboration with the European Respiratory Society (ERS). European Heart Journal 2020;41:543-603. DOI:10.1093/eurheartj/ehz405.

[47] Comerota AJ, Gale SS. Technique of contemporary iliofemoral and infrainguinal venous thrombectomy. J Vasc Surg 2006;43:185-91. DOI: 10.1016/j.jvs.2005.09.036.

[48] Muhlberger D, Wenkel M, PapapostolouG, Mumme A, Stucker M, Reich-Schupke S, et al. Surgical thrombectomy for iliofemoral deep vein thrombosis: Patient outcomes at 8.5 years. PLoS ONE 2020;15(6):e0235003. DOI: 10.1371/journal.pone.0235003.

Chapter 9

Mechanical Thrombectomy for Acute Pulmonary Ischemia

Adam Raskin, Anil Verma and Kofi Ansah

Abstract

Acute pulmonary embolism (PE) is a restrictive pulmonary vascular compromise with devastating complications depending on size and location. Massive and sub-massive classifications reflect hemodynamic compromise and cardiac dysfunction due to right ventricular strain, respectively. In addition to cardiac dysfunction, pulmonary ischemia and infarction play a key clinical factor. Mainstay management is with anticoagulation to prevent further clot propagation. Recent technological advances have revolutionized treatment modalities. Mechanical thrombectomy, catheter-based clot retrieval, is an effective way to eliminate emboli, restore cardiopulmonary function, and prevent ischemic injury. One such device, the FlowTriever System, has emerged as a way interventionalists can proceed with embolectomy and provide high level, life-saving care for acutely decompensated patients.

Keywords: pulmonary embolism, mechanical thrombectomy, FlowTriever

1. Introduction

Respiratory compromise due to embolization is one of the leading causes of death among hospitalized patients, a condition known as acute pulmonary embolism (PE). In the United States alone, for every 100,000 individuals, about 70 people will experience pulmonary embolism each calendar year [1].

Simply put, acute pulmonary embolism is a restriction of arterial blood flow in the lung that can be detrimental when misdiagnosed. When the cause of obstruction is blood itself, it is known as venous thromboembolism (VTE). This being the most common cause of pulmonary embolism. It is apropos to mention that blood flow is not the only substance that can cause mechanical lung obstructions. Other substances include, but not limited to fat (traumatic bone fracture, especially of long bones, leads to bone marrow/fat freely circulating systemically), amniotic fluid (as a complication of labor), air (a complication of central venous access), septic embolism (heart valve damage by micro-organism) or even tumor cells metastasizing. The broad array of materials that can lead to this obstructive shock makes it imperative for a clinician to put the clinical picture with the patient's symptoms to make the diagnosis early. Failure to do so in a timely manner can lead to catastrophic cardiopulmonary compromise and even death.

When PE is caused by venous thromboembolism, greater than 50% of patients will have some clot burden in their lower extremities or a deep vein thrombosis (DVT). The culprit vessels being the femoral and popliteal veins. Some patients may present with symptoms of DVT without PE. Therefore, a thorough investigation is warranted to diagnose, treat and prevent future propagation.

2. Pathophysiology of acute pulmonary embolism

Acute pulmonary embolism is a mechanical obstruction of the blood flow to the lung vasculature and the functional unit involved in respiration, the parenchyma. The parenchyma being starved of oxygen leads to an inflammatory response and cellular death made evident by respiratory compromise and the compensatory respiratory alkalosis on patient presentation. It is imperative to note that both PE and DVT share a spectrum in the realm of VTE. The main difference between these two disease states lies in the location. The main mechanism that leads to PE and DVT, known as the Virchow's triad, comprises of endothelial injury, venous statis and a hypercoagulable state.

Endothelial injury refers to damage to the vasculature which can lead to an inflammatory response in an attempt to heal with thrombus formation. Most commonly, this occurs in acute trauma, previous history of trauma or prior surgery. Venous stasis, which comprises of a no flow state of blood, can lead to thrombus formation as blood has an affinity to coagulate when not freely flowing. Venous stasis is mostly seen as a complication from immobility (postoperative states) or in patients with major strokes. Lastly, a hypercoagulable state can be a complication of disease states, such as active cancer, medications such as hormonal replacement therapy or oral contraceptives, and finally genetic mutations, most common being factor V Leiden. Other genetic mutations include: protein C and S deficiency, prothrombin gene mutation, antithrombin III deficiency.

Hemodynamically, there are many alterations that occur in the presence of an acute PE that is related to the size of the embolus, the duration of blood flow obstruction as well as the patient's cardiopulmonary history. Large PEs tend to obstruct the main pulmonary artery along with its branches while smaller PEs are culprits of the smaller peripheral vessels. The obstructive burden coupled with neurohormonal release contribute to hemodynamic compromise and ischemic propagation is presence of neurohormonal release that progress propagate ongoing damage. Common neurohormones present include serotonin, thrombin and histamine [2].

Hypoxic vasoconstriction, a reflex response to acute PE, leads to increase in mean arterial pulmonary pressure. This increase is significantly high in patients with history of pulmonary hypertension. Increased pulmonary artery pressure contributes to increased right ventricular (RV) afterload causing right ventricular enlargement and a leftward bulging of the interventricular septum commonly found on echocardiography. Cardiac arrest is hence from the vascular compromise from increased pressure on the right coronary artery, causing myocardial ischemia.

Acute PE impairs efficient gas exchange. Hypoxemia and increase in the alveolar-arterial oxygen tension gradient are the most common gas exchange abnormalities. Total dead space increases. Ventilation and perfusion become mismatched, with blood flow from obstructed pulmonary arteries redirected to other gas exchange units [2]. The obstruction of blood flow in the pulmonary arteries leads to a redistribution of blood flow causing some alveoli to have low ratios of ventilation to perfusion, whereas others have excessively high ratios of ventilation to perfusion [2].

3. Clinical manifestations

Assessment of PE in patients can be challenging as symptoms can be nonspecific. The patient could present with an array of different possibilities but a history of dyspnea, progressive or sudden onset in nature is a common complaint. Other complaints include pleuritic chest pain, cough and hemoptysis mostly in patients with pulmonary infarction. Due to the nonspecific symptoms that acute PE could present with, it is imperative to garner the appropriate risk factors that could lead to the suspicion. Another complaint that should increase the index of suspicion is a patient with dyspnea coupled with recent onset lower extremity tenderness or swelling.

Most patients with PE have tachypnea and tachycardia associated with hypoxemia. Similar findings can occur in disorders such as heart failure, pneumonia, or chronic obstructive pulmonary disease [2]. A good clinical examination is apropos to ascertain any other possible disease pathology that may mimic PE.

4. Diagnosis

The diagnosis of PE relies on a high clinical suspicion along with the patient's history and physical exam. After suspicion, confirmation with appropriate testing leads to the final diagnosis. Diagnostic tests alone are not the reflex course of action with a high index of suspicion due to the fact that there are many disease states that could present similarly. In patients with a high index of suspicion, the Wells criteria, developed by Wells et al., is a simple clinical model to predict the likelihood of PE. Scoring system has a maximum of 12.5 points, based on 7 variables: 3 points each for clinical evidence of DVT and an alternative diagnosis being less likely than PE, 1.5 points each for heart rate > 100 per minute, immobilization/surgery within 4 weeks, and previous deep vein thrombosis/PE, and 1 point each for hemoptysis or cancer [2, 3]. The pretest probability for PE after utilization of the Wells scoring system categorizes PE into low (score < 2), moderate (score between 2 and 6) or high risk (score > 6). This will then guide a clinician on subsequent tests such as a D-dimer assay, a byproduct of ineffective fibrinolysis released into systemic circulation. D-dimer elevation has high sensitivity for acute PE, as high as 98%, albeit poor sensitivity. Instances such as malignancy, advanced age and chronic inflammatory conditions are all reasons for an elevated d-dimer besides PE. Therefore, the benefit of a d-dimer assay lies in its high negative predictive value and its ability to effectively reduce further diagnostic testing in patients with an already low to moderate pretest probability with Wells scoring [4, 5].

Imaging studies in patients with acute PE in recent times have been with computed tomography pulmonary angiography (CT-PA). The benefit of CT-PA is direct thrombi visualization in the pulmonary arteries and effectively ruling out patients without PE [2]. The use of radiocontrast dye should be taken into consideration in patients with a suspicion of PE, but in patients with decompensation coupled with a high index of suspicion, the benefits of imaging clearly outweigh the risk. Furthermore, CT-PA with evidence of thrombus in the pulmonary arteries up to the segmental level provides strong evidence of PE. When negative, it does exclude PE but the presence of PE in the subsegmental regions, sometimes missed by CT-PA, does not alter patient outcome as these patients have at least as good an outcome as patients with a negative lung scan [2, 6].

There are indeed other modalities for investigation of acute PE, though by far a CT-PA has emerged as the more favorable option. Other modalities include a ventilation-perfusion (V/Q) scan, a two-part exam with a ventilation phase and perfusion phase. Diagnosis of PE based on a V/Q scan is made when PE-associated lung areas fail to enhance on the perfusion phase using technetium-labeled albumin macroaggregates. Magnetic resonance imaging (MRI) with gadolinium-enhancement has been shown to have similar efficacy to that of CT-PA.

5. Management of acute pulmonary embolism

Anticoagulation has become the mainstay treatment for acute PE though the degree of severity influences the length of treatment. The severity of acute PE depends on parameters such as hemodynamics, right ventricular dysfunction, presence of troponin and/or brain natriuretic peptide (BNP). Risk stratification using the appropriate criteria not only guides the choice of treatment, but also provides outpatient management options. It is also highly important to know if the patient has any contraindications to anticoagulation prior to initiation of treatment. Massive (high-risk) PE is the presence of hemodynamic compromise, right ventricular dysfunction and increased troponin and/or BNP levels. In such patients, the most common cause of death is not the PE, but the complication of acute right ventricular failure. To mitigate this complication, hemodynamic and respiratory support early is crucial. Due to the dependence of preload in right ventricular failure, both fluid expansion and inotropic agents, such as dobutamine, dopamine and/or norepinephrine, are needed to manage shock [2]. In patients with presence of right ventricular dysfunction and increased troponin and/or BNP levels without hemodynamic compromise, are classified as sub-massive (intermediate-risk) PE with consideration of fibrinolytic therapy if very symptomatic. Lastly, low-risk PE classification is in the group of patients with no hemodynamic compromise, right ventricular dysfunction or increased troponin or BNP levels. In such patients, a consideration of outpatient management is acceptable.

5.1 Anticoagulation

Anticoagulation has become the cornerstone modality of treatment in patients with acute PE. In patients with a very high index of suspicion or massive PE, anticoagulation should be initiated prior to confirmatory test. The most extensively studied anticoagulant in PE is heparin. Heparin, an anti-thrombin III inhibitor, acts mainly by inactivation of factor Xa in the clotting cascade, preventing the conversion of prothrombin to thrombin. Other options include low molecular weight heparin (LMWH), fondaparinux or the direct factor Xa inhibitors, rivaroxaban and apixaban. Dosing for heparin is usually 80 U/kg bolus followed by an infusion at the rate of 18 U/kg per hour with subsequent doses based on aPTT results [4]. Additionally, it is important to monitor platelet count while heparin is administered due to the risk of heparin-induced thrombocytopenia (HIT). After the initial heparinization phase, continued treatment is with an oral direct thrombin inhibitor, factor Xa inhibitor or warfarin.

The duration of treatment of PE is directly related to the precipitating factors that led to the PE. In other words, whether the PE was provoked or unprovoked. Special considerations in terms of treatment modality and duration are made for certain populations such as pregnant females or patients with active cancer. For all other patient populations with who present with a first time PE, the minimum duration of treatment is 3 months. If the PE is provoked and the factors are withdrawn such as a female stopping hormonal treatment, then a 3-month period of oral anticoagulation is sufficient. In patients with an unprovoked or life-threatening PE, indefinite anticoagulation is ideal due to a higher risk of recurrence. There must be a risk and benefit analysis when indefinite anticoagulation is being pursued, especially in patients with a higher bleeding risk [4].

5.2 Thrombolytic therapy

Systemic thrombolytic therapy is an effective therapy in preventing deaths from PE, however it markedly increases bleeding risks, including intracranial and fatal bleeding [7]. The PEITHO (Pulmonary Embolism Thrombolysis Study), which compared tenecteplase with placebo in 1000 PE patients without hypotension but with right ventricular dysfunction, found no clear net benefit from systemic thrombolytic therapy; the reduction in cardiovascular collapse (odds ratio: 0.30) was offset by the increase in major bleeding (odds ratio: 5.2) [8]. Consequently, systemic thrombolytic therapy is usually reserved for PE patients with hypotension. Catheter-directed thrombolysis (CDT) was initially developed for treatment of arterial, dialysis graft, and deep vein thromboses (leg or arm). When used to treat acute PE, a wire is usually passed through the embolus, followed by placement of a multi-sidehole infusion catheter through which a thrombolytic drug is infused over 12–24 h. The delivery of the drug directly into the thrombus is expected to be as effective as systemic therapy but to cause less bleeding because a much lower dose of the drug is used.

SEATTLE II is a single-arm prospective cohort study in which 150 patients with lobar artery or more central PE (31 with and 119 without hypotension) were treated with ultrasound-assisted CDT using a standardized protocol [9]. Tissue plasminogen activator was infused into each treated lung at a rate of 1 mg/h, to a total dose of 24 mg (over 12 h for bilateral lung infusions), and no additional mechanical maneuvers were used to disrupt or aspirate thrombus. When computed tomography pulmonary angiography was repeated after 48 h, the right ventricular to left ventricular ratio was decreased by 27% and thrombus burden was reduced by 30%. Pulmonary artery pressure also decreased by 27% between the start to the end of CDT. These 3 improvements were each highly statistically significant. There were 17 episodes of major bleeding in 15 patients (10%): one was associated with hypotension; all required transfusion; none was intracranial; and none was fatal.

5.3 Mechanical thrombectomy

Acute pulmonary ischemia due to pulmonary embolism results in a cascade of events, from decreasing lung compliance to increasing pulmonary resistance ultimately resulting in RV dysfunction and hemodynamic collapse. Thus, in certain cases more rapid thrombus removal is required, and mechanical techniques are now available.

The FlowTriever System (**Figure 1**) is a mechanical thrombectomy device indicated for use in the peripheral vasculature and pulmonary arteries (PAs). FlowTriever received U.S. Food and Drug Administration 510(k) clearance for PE in May 2018—the first mechanical thrombectomy device to receive that indication. The FlowTriever System includes Triever aspiration catheters (16-F, 20-F, 24-F) capable of removing large amounts of thrombus via aspiration with a 60 cc syringe. The FlowTriever System also includes FlowTriever catheters with three

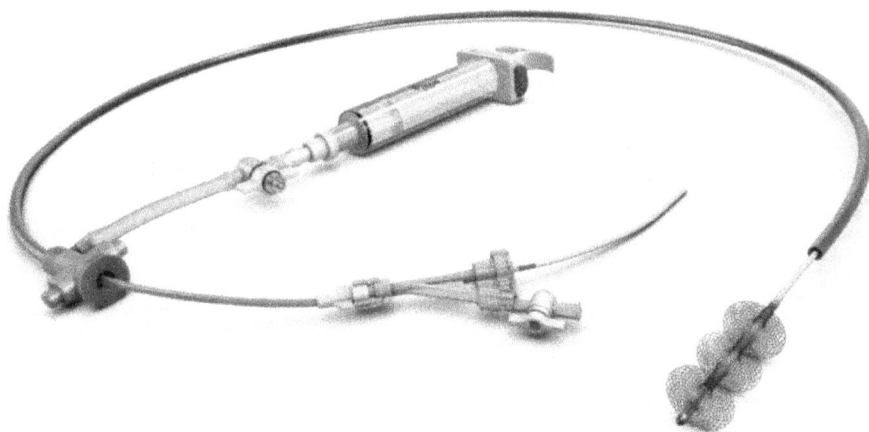

Figure 1.
The FlowTriever® system. The Triever aspiration catheter is shown in purple, and the optional FlowTriever® catheter with nitinol disks is shown emerging from the distal end of the Triever catheter.

self-expanding nitinol mesh disks of different sizes designed to aid in extraction, if needed, by engaging and disrupting thrombus. Anticoagulation with heparin is recommended per routine catheterization laboratory practice to prevent thrombosis of the catheter. The aspiration catheter is advanced over a 0.035-inch wire to the level of the right or left PA, just proximal to the occlusive thrombus. Once engaged, the clot is extracted via aspiration through the catheter. The procedure can be repeated several times per side at the discretion of the physician, depending on the amount of clot retrieved and the improvement in distal flow on repeat angiography.

The FlowTriever System has been evaluated in several clinical studies both prospectively and retrospectively. The first of these was a prospective multi-center study, the FLARE (FlowTriever Pulmonary Embolectomy Clinical Study) trial, which was the largest systematic evaluation of the effectiveness of mechanical thrombectomy for PE at the time [10]. From April 2016 to October 2017, 106 patients were treated with the FlowTriever System at 18 U.S. sites. Two patients (1.9%) received adjunctive thrombolytics. The mean procedural time was 94 min, and the mean intensive care unit stay was 1.5 days. Forty-three patients (41.3%) did not require any intensive care unit stay. At 48 h post-procedure, average RV/LV ratio reduction was 0.38 (25.1%; $p < 0.0001$). Four patients (3.8%) experienced 6 major adverse events, with 1 patient (1.0%) experiencing major bleeding. One patient (1.0%) died from undiagnosed breast cancer through 30-day follow-up. The trial concluded that percutaneous mechanical thrombectomy with the FlowTriever System appears safe and effective in patients with acute intermediate-risk PE, achieved significant improvement in RV/LV ratio, and resulted in minimal major bleeding.

Large-bore aspiration mechanical thrombectomy with the FlowTriever System was also evaluated in two retrospective single-arm clinical studies. The first of these [11] was a single-center study of 46 patients with both massive (high-risk) and submassive (intermediate-risk) PE. The authors reported a significant reduction in mean PA pressure from 33.9 ± 8.9 mmHg to 27.0 ± 9.0 mmHg ($p < 0.0001$) immediately following thrombectomy. The majority of patients experienced intraprocedural reductions in mean PA pressure (88%) and supplemental oxygen requirements (71%). All patients survived to discharge, and there were no procedure-related complications or deaths within the 30 days following discharge. The second retrospective study [12] was a multi-center study of 34 patients with massive and very-high-risk submassive PE. All patients were either hemodynamically unstable, intubated, or normotensive but with low cardiac index (< 1.8 L/min/m^2). In this very sick population, cardiac index improved significantly immediately following thrombectomy (2.0 ± 0.1 L/min/m^2 vs. 2.4 ± 0.1 L/min/m^2, $p = 0.1$), as did mean PA pressure (33.2 ± 1.6 mmHg vs. 25.0 ± 1.5 mmHg, $p = .01$). Two patients deteriorated during the procedure, one who expired and one who was stabilized on ECMO. All other patients survived through a mean follow-up of 205 days. These two retrospective studies provide clinical evidence supporting the safety and effectiveness of mechanical thrombectomy with the FlowTriever System for PE treatment.

More recently, the FlowTriever System was studied in a nonrandomized two-arm retrospective analysis versus routine care [13]. This single-center study compared outcomes for 28 patients who underwent mechanical thrombectomy with the FlowTriever System to those for 30 patients who received routine care, which consisted of anticoagulation alone, anticoagulation with CDT, or systemic thrombolysis. In-hospital mortality was significantly lower for patients undergoing mechanical thrombectomy versus routine care (3.6% vs. 23.3%, $p < 0.05$). Furthermore, the average intensive care unit length of stay was also significantly shorter for patients undergoing mechanical thrombectomy (2.1 ± 1.2 days vs. 6.1 ± 8.6 days, $p < 0.05$). Total hospital length of stay and 30-day readmission rates were similar between the two groups. This study provides initial comparative data suggesting that mechanical thrombectomy can improve in-hospital mortality and decrease ICU length of stay for PE patients with elevated risk profiles.

5.4 Technical aspects of mechanical thrombectomy

1. Pre procedure planning

   a. Patient Information

      i. Prior to any pulmonary embolism procedure several patient conditions must be made clear. Several questions that all operators should ask include, what are the current hemodynamics and does that patient require vasopressor support? What is the current respiratory status (Ie O2 supplementation or on mechanical ventilation)? What is the bleeding risk and can the patient be anticoagulated? During our procedure we maintain and actual clotting time (ACT) of >250 secs.

   b. Pre case Imaging

      i. CT is the most rapid and common imaging tool used. Specific items to look for include, location and size of clot, RV/LV Ratio, and pulmonary infarct.

      ii. Echocardiography will not only show LV and RV size but RV systolic function.

   c. Additional things to consider:

      i. History or current DVT

      ii. IVC Filter in Place

        iii. Clot in Transit (is TEE or TTE available urgently)

        iv. Recent Surgery/Extended immobile time (travel)

        v. Cancer History

        vi. History of PE

        vii. Infarct consideration (reperfusion injury/elevated wire perforation risk)

    d. Anesthesia:

        i. Conscious sedation is recommended. General Anesthesia has a risk of worsening hypotension and reducing preload to the RV. If systemic pressure is tenuous, a rapid reduction in RV filling can result in immediate hemodynamic collapse.

2. Patient Selection

    a. Avoidance of thrombolytics

        i. There are several advantages to the decision making for who would benefit from thrombolytic therapy for pulmonary embolism. The immediate decision is to determine who is at highest risk and thus has the largest to gain. Any patient with right ventricular (RV) dysfunction, we feel should be considered for thrombolytic therapy. Patients with an elevated RV: LV ratio; greater than 0.9, elevated pro-bnp, elevated troponins, and hemodynamics suggestive of reduced cardiac output, should be considered for thrombolytic therapy.

        ii. Patients need to be able to lay either supine or prone for a minimum of 30 minutes, thus taking oxygen requirements and body habitus into consideration.

        iii. Any patient with a relative contraindication to thrombolytic therapy, or felt to be at elevated risk, immediately should be considered for thrombotic intervention.

3. Access

    a. US guidance

        i. Access to venous circulation, when using large bore sheaths should always be performed with ultrasound guidance. It is advantageous in the venous system to evaluate for upper or lower extremity deep venous thrombosis, prior to starting the procedure, as well as avoidance of an arterial puncture.

    b. Femoral

        i. The most common access site for pulmonary thrombectomy is the common femoral vein

    c. Jugular

        i. When an alternative access is required another option is the internal jugular vein.

4. Pulmonary angiogram

    a. Difficulties

        i. Image quality tends to be the dis-advantage. Morbid obesity, patient movement, as well as variations in imaging acquisition (ie dye load, manual vs. power injection), can result in wide range of image quality.

5. Aspiration thrombectomy catheters

    a. Inari Medical

        i. Twenty-four french aspiration guide catheter that navigates through the right heart and delivers the catheter directly into the pulmonary artery. Aspiration is performed by a manual pull. The large bore catheter maximizes aspiration and collection of thrombus. The 24 F catheter creates an aspiration flow rate of 143 mLs/second.

        ii. Sixteen french curve

            1. Due to the natural curvature of the pulmonary artery to the right, the 24 F catheter takes a turn to the right pulmonary artery typically with little difficulty. The catheter when placed in the left pulmonary artery, typically does not engage the left lower lobe. The 16 french curve catheter is placed within the 24F catheter and is preshaped to point down into the left pulmonary artery for selective thrombus aspiration.

        iii. Bloodloss technology

            1. The FlowSaver blood return system is designed to be used with the FlowTriever aspiration catheter to reduced blood loss by filtering aspirated thrombi and blood for reinfusion back to the patient, thus enabling bloodless thrombectomy for pulmonary embolism procedure. The filtration system includes a 40-micro filter. Filtered blood can be reintroduced using a 60-cc collection syringe.

    b. Penumbra, Inc.

        i. The Indigo aspiration system is indicated for use in the peripheral arterial system and the pulmonary arteries, receiving U.S. Food and Drug Administration 510(k) clearance for PE in December 2019.

ii. The Indigo system lightning 12 aspiration catheter that navigates through the right heart and into the selected pulmonary artery. The 12F system, unlike the manual aspiration of the Inari device, is connected to the Penumbra aspiration pump, resulting in a continuous vacuum system at -28.5 mmHg. If thrombus is not aspirated, the system also has a separator wire that can be advanced through the catheter to disrupt thrombus at the distal tip.

6. Intraprocedural complications

    a. Perforation

        i. The most common cause of pulmonary artery perforation is due to a wire complication. Wire perforation causes include treating distal clot, poor wire positioning and overlapping vessel (specifically on the left side)

        ii. Avoidance and Management

            1. Limit use of guide wires, and always use Amplatz wire to work over

            2. Use multiple shots to confirm location of wire and catheter

            3. Use multiple angles of monitor to confirm locations

            4. If Perforation does occur, increase supplemental oxygen, stop and reverse anticoagulation and consider placing a occlusion balloon proximal to the perforation.

    b. Right heart trauma

        i. If the tricuspid valve crossed safely with angled pigtail catheter or balloon tip catheter, typically not as concerned. If a end hold catheter was used, through a chordae tendinea of the tricuspid valve.

        ii. Always advance with caution as advancing through heart monitoring pain, excessive tension advancing catheter, and any arrhythmias happening

        iii. Never advance large bore catheters without dilators

        iv. Use buddy wires to assist stability in accessing multiple vessels to avoid kick back

    c. Shock/RV failure

        i. There are several methods of determining right ventricular systolic function. A calculated PAPi in the cardiac cath lab can determine who would benefit from RV mechanical support (ie Abiomed Impella RP). If the PAPi is calculated to be less than 1, and you have achieved enough thrombolytic therapy to allow for distal perfusion, mechanical support should be considered. Extracorporeal membrane oxygenation (ECMO) can also be considered for both hemodynamic support and oxygenation.

7. Closure

   a. Most venous access sites can be closed with manual pressure alone. However, with large bore access we have using the Abbott Medical proglide perclose suture mediated closure. This device has been shown to reduce time to hemostasis, ambulation and discharge compared to manual compression

8. Post Procedure management

   a. ICU avoidance

      i. The use of thrombolysis for the treatment of PE at some institutions requires ICU level care.

      ii. Mechanical thrombectomy is a means of direct therapy which can result in immediate clinical response and will commonly not require intensive care management.

      iii. Additionally with the avoidance of tissue plasminogen activator (tPA), ICU admission post procedure is commonly unnecessary.

   b. Venous dopplers

      i. The most common source of PE is DVT. Thus, all patients require bilateral venous duplex for confirmation of residual disease.

      ii. Based on these results, it is a clinical decision whether therapy is required for DVT.

   c. Hypercoagulable work up

      i. Patients who benefit from this work up include:

         • those with/without a family history of VTE

         • patients age < 45 years

         • recurrent thrombosis or thrombosis in unusual sites

         • arterial thrombosis

         • history of warfarin-induced dermatologic necrosis

      ii. These patients will benefit from testing: activated protein C resistance, factor V Leiden, Prothrombin gene mutation, Protein C and S deficiency, Antithrombin deficiency.

d. DOAC

    i. DOACS such as Factor Xa inhibitors, Apixaban or Rivaroxaban, have become more favorable than Warfarin for anticoagulation due to lower bleeding risk, monitoring for therapeutic INR levels and easier dosing. Apixaban is dosed twice daily while Rivaroxaban is daily dosing. A lower dose is required based on age ≥80, weight ≤60kg and creatinine ≥1.5

e. Follow up Echo

    i. A follow up echo is used to determine RV dimensions, RV dysfunction and residual pulmonary hypertension.

    ii. It is our practice that if there is residual elevation of pulmonary systolic pressure, we refer the patient to a pulmonary hypertension specialist.

5.5 Mechanical thrombectomy case reports

- Case 1

  o A 33-year-old woman with no significant past medical history presented to our emergency department after multiple syncopal episodes. An ambulance service was called by family and the patient arrived hypotensive and poorly responsive. She required 6 L of supplemental oxygen and vasopressor support to keep a mean arterial pressure greater than 60 mmHg and oxygen saturation greater than 92%. A bedside anterior-posterior chest X-ray showed a normal cardiac silhouette and clear lung fields. A 12-lead electrocardiogram was consistent with a sinus tachycardia and right bundle branch block. Initial laboratory data was positive for an elevated d-dimer (> 5000 ng/mL), positive troponin (0.4 ng/mL), and pro-brain natriuretic peptide (> 10,000 pg/mL). A stat CT angiogram of the chest demonstrated a massive PE with complete occlusion of the left lower lobe and a RV/LV ratio of 1.5.

  o The patient was moved emergently to the cardiac catheterization laboratory for immediate therapeutic aspiration thrombectomy. Access was obtained in the right femoral vein using ultrasound guidance. Initial systolic PA pressure was 60 mmHg and the mean PA pressure was 35 mmHg. A pulmonary angiogram confirmed complete occlusion of the left lower lobe (**Figure 2**). The 24-F Triever aspiration catheter (Triever24) was positioned in the left pulmonary artery. A 20-F Triever Curve catheter, capable of curving up to 260° to aid in navigating in difficult anatomies, (**Figure 3**) was used coaxially with the Triever24 catheter to angle to the lower lobe where two aspirations were performed. A large amount of thrombus was removed (**Figure 4**) and repeat pulmonary angiography showed almost complete pulmonary artery opacification and large reduction in thrombus burden (**Figure 5**). Within minutes there was hemodynamic improvement and oxygen requirements returned to room air alone. Post-thrombectomy pulmonary artery systolic pressure was 33 mmHg. The patient was transferred to the general medical ward and started on oral Factor Xa inhibitor and discharged home the following day.

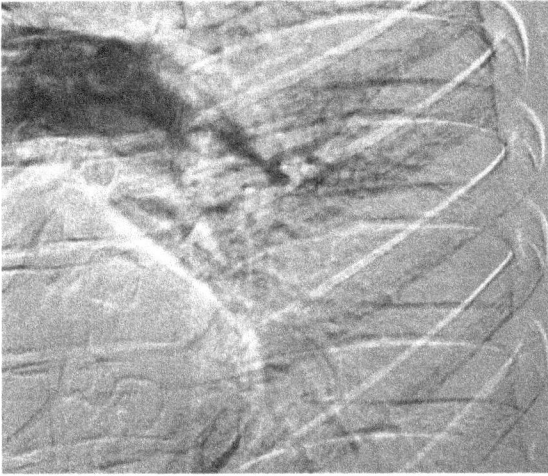

Figure 2.
Pre-treatment pulmonary angiogram showing complete occlusion of the left lower lobe in a patient with massive pulmonary embolism.

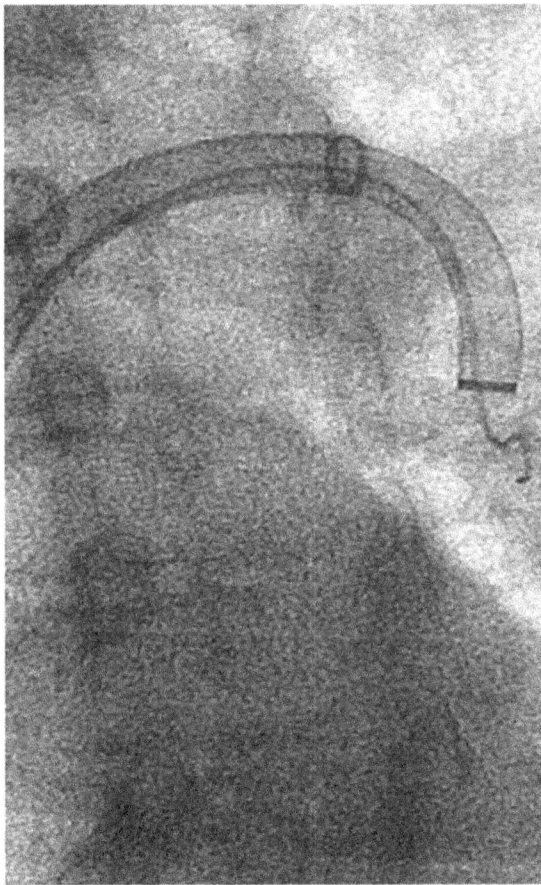

Figure 3.
Intra-procedure pulmonary angiogram showing the Triever20 curve catheter coaxial within the larger Triever24 catheter in the left lower lobe of the lung in a PE patient.

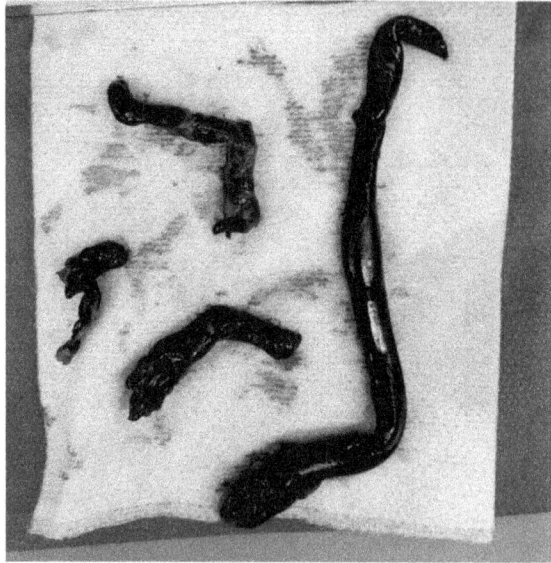

Figure 4.
A large amount of thrombus extracted with the FlowTriever® system from a PE patient.

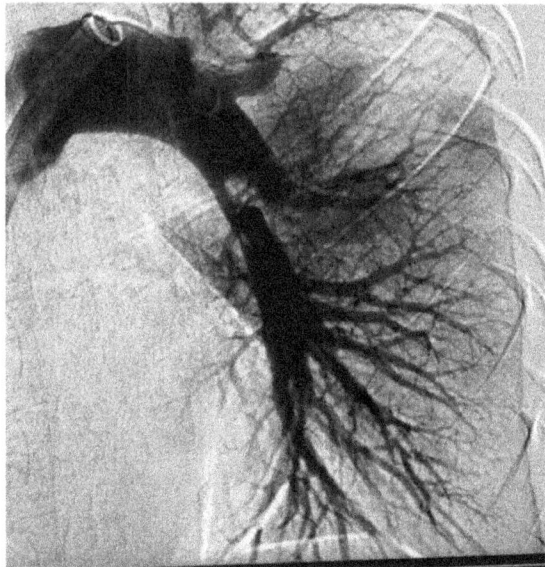

Figure 5.
Post-thrombectomy pulmonary angiogram showing almost complete pulmonary artery opacification and large reduction in thrombus burden.

- Case 2

    o A 75-year-old man with a past medical history of metastatic prostate cancer with known spinal involvement, presented to our emergency room with acute onset of shortness of breath and chest tightness. Initial oxygen saturation was 82% requiring high flow oxygen with a non-rebreather mask. Initial blood pressure was 110/80 mmHg and heart rate of 110 bpm.

The pretest probability of PE was high thus the first diagnostic test was a CT pulmonary angiogram, which confirmed a saddle pulmonary embolism and large thrombus burden in the left and right lobes. The RV/LV ratio was 1.4.

○ Pulmonary angiography was consistent with CT findings (**Figure 6**). With a known history of spinal metastasis, thrombolytic therapy was contraindicated. The femoral vein access site was dilated to accommodate a 24-F sheath, the Flowtriever System was positioned into the mainstem pulmonary artery and a single aspiration was performed. The catheter was

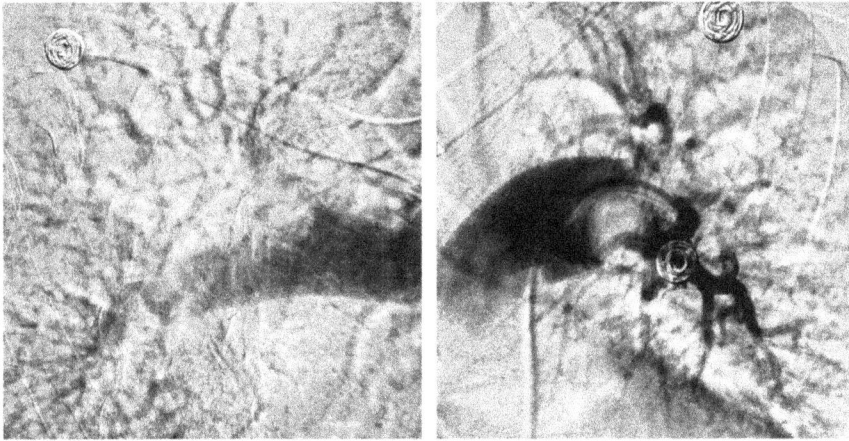

Figure 6.
Pre-thrombectomy pulmonary angiography of the right and left lungs demonstrating a saddle pulmonary embolism with large thrombus burden.

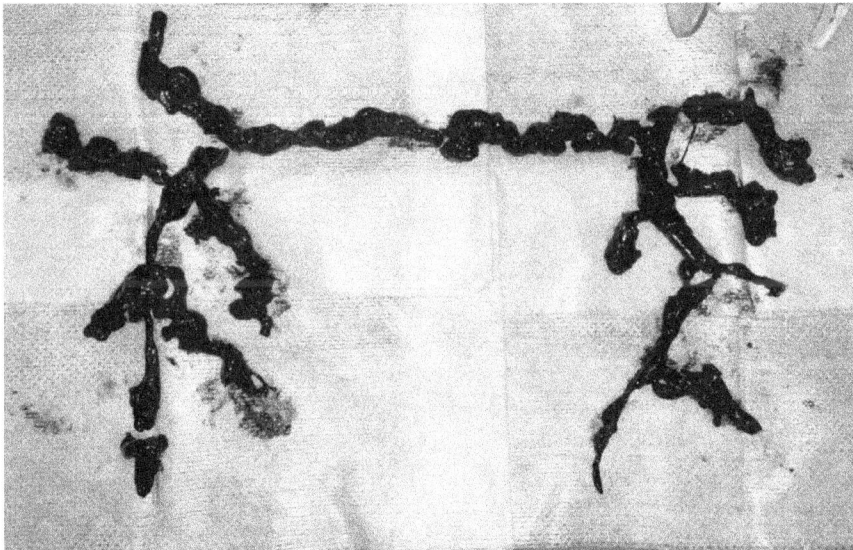

Figure 7.
Thrombus extracted using the FlowTriever® system.

then positioned into the left pulmonary artery performing a single aspiration, followed by the right pulmonary artery, again requiring a single aspiration. Repeat angiography confirmed thrombus resolution and large clot removal (**Figure** 7). The patient was transferred to the general medical floor on room air. An echocardiogram performed the next day demonstrated normal right ventricular size and function with normal pulmonary pressures. The patient was discharged home the following day.

- Case 3

  o A 44-year-old woman with a recent history of COVID-19 pneumonia presented from home with acute worsening of dyspnea and new pleuritic chest pain. Prior to this admission she required no supplemental oxygen,

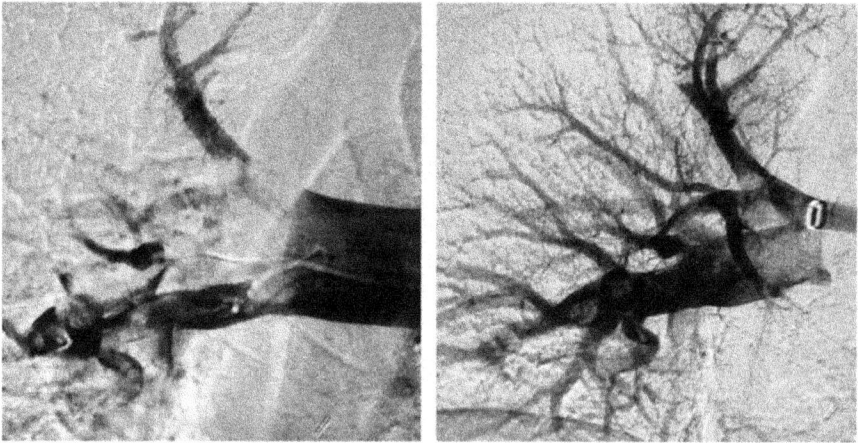

Figure 8.
Pre- (left) and post-thrombectomy (right) pulmonary angiograms demonstrating large thrombus burden prior to thrombectomy with the FlowTriever® system and subsequent resolution post-thrombectomy.

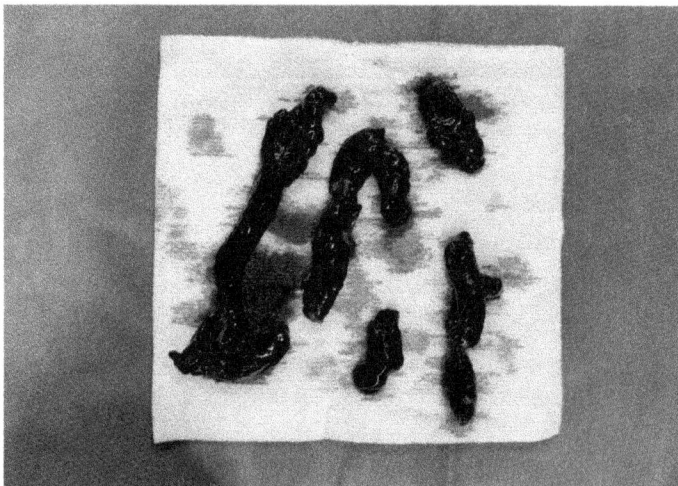

Figure 9.
Large amount of thrombus extracted with the FlowTriever® system in a patient with history of COVID-19.

however, now was on 10 L of oxygen to maintain a saturation > 96%. A CT angiogram of the chest was consistent with a massive right middle lobe pulmonary embolism. The patient was taken to the cardiac catheterization laboratory for emergent intervention. Due to rapid decline in respiratory status and acute hypoxic respiratory failure, the patient was placed on mechanical ventilation. In order to provide rapid therapy, aspiration thrombectomy was performed in the right pulmonary artery. Initial pulmonary angiogram clearly demonstrated large thrombus burden of the right pulmonary artery (**Figure 8**, left). After a single aspiration was performed, repeat angiogram confirmed almost complete resolution (**Figure 8**, right), and large thrombus debulking (**Figure 9**). At the conclusion of the procedure, the patient required <40% fraction of inspired oxygen (Fio2) and positive end-expiratory pressure (PEEP) of 5, maintaining an oxygen saturation > 99%. That evening while in the intensive care unit she was successfully extubated and required 2 L of oxygen by nasal cannula. Seventy-two hours after her initial presentation, she was discharged home on room air.

Author details

Adam Raskin[1], Anil Verma[1] and Kofi Ansah[2*]

1 Mercy Heart Institute, Mercy West Hospital, Cincinnati, Ohio, USA

2 Jewish Hospital, Cincinnati, Ohio, USA

*Address all correspondence to: knansah@mercy.com

IntechOpen

References

[1] Papadakis MA, McPhee SJ, Rabow MW. Current Medical Diagnosis & Treatment 2020: Pulmonary Disorders. 59th ed. New York: McGraw-Hill Education; 2019. pp. 308-315

[2] Goldhaber SZ, Elliott CG. Acute pulmonary embolism: Part I: Epidemiology, pathophysiology, and diagnosis. Circulation. 2003;**108**(22): 2726-2729

[3] Wells PS, Anderson DR, Rodger M, Ginsberg JS, Kearon C, Gent M, et al. Derivation of a simple clinical model to categorize patients probability of pulmonary embolism: Increasing the models utility with the SimpliRED D-dimer. Thrombosis and Haemostasis. 2000;**83**(03):416-420

[4] Goldman L, Schafer AI. Goldman-Cecil Medicine: Pulmonary Embolism. 25th ed. Amsterdam: Elsevier; 2015. pp. 620-626

[5] Huisman MV, Klok FA. Diagnostic management of acute deep vein thrombosis and pulmonary embolism. Journal of Thrombosis and Haemostasis. 2013;**11**(3):412-422

[6] Anderson DR, Kahn SR, Rodger MA, Kovacs MJ, Morris T, Hirsch A, et al. Computed tomographic pulmonary angiography vs ventilation-perfusion lung scanning in patients with suspected pulmonary embolism: A randomized controlled trial. Journal of the American Medical Association. 2007;**298**(23): 2743-2753

[7] Chatterjee S, Chakraborty A, Weinberg I, Kadakia M, Wilensky RL, Sardar P, et al. Thrombolysis for pulmonary embolism and risk of all-cause mortality, major bleeding, and intracranial hemorrhage: A meta-analysis. Journal of the American Medical Association. 2014;**311**(23): 2414-2421

[8] Meyer G, Vicaut E, Danays T, Agnelli G, Becattini C, Beyer-Westendorf J, et al. Fibrinolysis for patients with intermediate-risk pulmonary embolism. The New England Journal of Medicine. 2014;**370**: 1402-1411

[9] Piazza G, Hohlfelder B, Jaff MR, Ouriel K, Engelhardt TC, Sterling KM, et al. A prospective, single-arm, multicenter trial of ultrasound-facilitated, catheter-directed, low-dose fibrinolysis for acute massive and submassive pulmonary embolism: The SEATTLE II study. Cardiovascular Interventions. 2015;**8**(10):1382-1392

[10] Tu T, Toma C, Tapson VF, Adams C, Jaber WA, Silver M, et al. A prospective, single-arm, multicenter trial of catheter-directed mechanical thrombectomy for intermediate-risk acute pulmonary embolism: The FLARE study. JACC. Cardiovascular Interventions. 2019;**12**(9):859-869

[11] Wible BC, Buckley JR, Cho KH, Bunte MC, Saucier NA, Borsa JJ. Safety and efficacy of acute pulmonary embolism treated via large-bore aspiration mechanical thrombectomy using the Inari FlowTriever device. Journal of Vascular and Interventional Radiology. 2019;**30**(9):1370-1375

[12] Toma C, Khandhar S, Zalewski AM, D'Auria SJ, Tu TM, Jaber WA. Percutaneous thrombectomy in patients with massive and very high-risk submassive acute pulmonary embolism. Catheterization and Cardiovascular Interventions. 2020;**96**(7):1465-1470

[13] Buckley JR, Wible BC. In-hospital mortality and related outcomes for elevated risk acute pulmonary embolism treated with mechanical thrombectomy versus routine care. Journal of Intensive Care Medicine. 2021:088506662110 36446